TRIBAL STUDIES OF INDIA SERIES T 186

PUTTING PEOPLE LAST
TRIBAL DISPLACEMENT AND REHABILITATION

TRIBAL STUDIES OF INDIA SERIES T 186

PUTTING PEOPLE LAST

TRIBAL DISPLACEMENT AND REHABILITATION

H.S. Saksena
Chandra Sen

INTER-INDIA PUBLICATIONS
D-17, Raja Garden, New Delhi-110015 (India)
Phone: 91-11-5441120, Telefax: 91-11-5467082
e-mail: interinp@ndb.vsnl.net.in

ISBN 81-210-0390-3

First Published in India in 1999

ISBN 81-210-0390-3
9 788121 003902

Printed and Published in India by :
M.C. MITTAL
INTER-INDIA PUBLICATIONS
(PRINTERS AND PUBLISHERS)
D-17 RAJA GARDEN
NEW DELHI-110015 (INDIA)
Phone : 91-11-5441120 Telefax : 91-11-5467082
e.mail : interinp@ndb.vsnl.net.in

Dedicated to the Memory
of
Professor D.N. Majumdar

Our

Ever Inspiring Teacher

FOREWORD

It is a privilege to write a foreword to a study by knowledgeable and socially sensitive scholars like H.S. Saksena and Chandra Sen on displacement and rehabilitation of tribal and scheduled caste population in Sonbhadra district, Uttar Pradesh.

The study relates to the impact of setting up of a number of irrigation, power and mining projects in Sonbhadra district. The researchers have, however, succeeded to present the study in a wider canvas by referring to overall picture of displacement and rehabilitation caused by different types of development projects in the country; step by step unfolding the policy frames adopted by various agencies at the state, national and international levels in dealing with the problems of the project affected persons; the extent of implementation of the policy guidelines; the overall pattern visible in the functioning of the implementing agencies and the responses of the affected populations at individual and collective levels articulated in their verbal statements and action.

The study covers six major projects, namely, Rihand Reservoir, Singrauli Super-Thermal Power Station, Anpara Thermal Power Station, NCL Coalfields at Kakri, Bina and Khadia, Rihand Nagar Super Thermal Power Project and Kanhar Irrigation Project. It is based on field enquiries as well as examination of secondary source materials. A schedule was canvassed among 1038 families, roughly 10 percent of the oustee families. In addition autobiographies of 31 persons were recorded. Project level data were collected through a brief questionnaire. It was followed by interviews with concerned officers, prominent functionaries of NGOs operating in the area and other knowledgeable persons. Secondary source materials include the Land Acquisition Act 1894 and its amendment in 1984; the Coal Bearing Areas (Acquisition and Development) Act, 1957; Policy Statement of the Ministry of Water Resources, Ministry of Home Affairs, Bureau of Public Enterprises, Government of Uttar Pradesh, Northern Coal Fields Limited (NCL), National Thermal Power Corporation (NTPC), and the World Bank. The report also includes Supreme Court's Directives in a Public Interest Litigation initiated by the Banaswasi Sewa Asram, relevant to tribal lands, some of which were acquired by NTPC. The report gives useful insights about the complicated nature of the problem by drawing upon several other sources.

Certainly the research study with its lucid descriptive accounts underpinned by relevant statistical data as well as an analytical account of the leadership issues in the caste-tribal communities in this remote area will provide useful reference material for those currently interested in the problems of those who are described as project affected persons.

But the real strong point of the work goes much beyond this limited purpose. Through the biographical narrations of 31 persons, the report has projected an informed story of bleeding souls of individuals and communities. It poses a challenge not only to the votaries of 'new temples', as Jawaharlal Nehru described one such project, but also to the countrymen in general. In the name of development a great human tragedy is taking place, ironically lauded by a myth of great achievement.

The tragedy is two faceted. One facet of it is obvious. Thousands of families have become homeless, thousands of persons have become jobless, hundreds of village communities have become disrupted, dozens of ethnic entities have lost their moorings in space. One of the project evictees has described the rehabilitation colony as *mrityulok* (land of death).

But the greater tragedy is that it is not one colony or similar colonies sprouting up in the wake of the mega-projects operating in India or even in other parts of the world, which mark the dotted lands of death; the whole world has perhaps turned into a planet of living death. Today it is spiritual death; tomorrow it may as well be physical death.

When a senior functionary of a project claims to have 'civilized' the people or howls on the face of human misery, 'it's very good of the government to pay you anything' 'that's good enough for yokels like you', he is either spiritually dead or is wallowing in his dehumanised animus. There are many more like him. They are not only in India; they are all over the globe. But they themselves are victims of pernicious world system. Utter cynicism with which 'development' projects are being implemented in countries of Latin America, Africa, Asia or even in North America and Scandinavian countries of Europe (in so far as the indigenous peoples of the last two continents are concerned) reveal the bottom of human degradation. If one adds to the same the pollutants created all over the world in the pursuit of political power and endless greed, one may not be unjustified to envisage that the 21st century will be the last century of human presence on the planet. The utter indifference with which bulk of the peoples in India and in other parts of the world are allowing not only the human meaning of their existence, but even their physical survival to be mortgaged to the worship of Mannon, shows that mankind as a whole has become spiritually benumbed.

There are certainly sensitive individuals and institutions even today who are trying to avert the disaster. Some of the policy guidelines described here in detail is an affirmation of the same. But then one is to reflect why they are hardly implemented anywhere. It would not be correct to question the sincerity of the persons who formulate the guidelines. It will also not be correct to indict in isolation the functionaries who fail to implement the guidelines. It is the over-all political-economic environment which is to be taken into consideration. Trans-national corporate bodies have now emerged as superstates. They have functional autonomy of their own. Humanity, humanism are anathema to them. Individuals do not matter. It is the imperative of the system that matters.

The genii has been released. The guidelines are the attempts to bottle up the genii. These are needed. By describing and discussing them in detail in the study the researchers have done a yeomen service. The critical flaw with the guidelines is that these do not touch some of the basic questions. One of the basic questions is the legal epistemology relating to land and land based property. As a legacy Anglo-saxon legal system the concepts of *res nullius* (land that has not been assigned by sovereign belongs to the sovereign) and *terra nullius* (land to which human labour is not visibly perceived as an input is nobody's land and hence state has the prime claim over such land) prevail almost all over the world. These concepts are now being challenged in some countries including India. Much of the failure of the implementing agencies of the development projects and project affected persons' rehabilitation programmes can be traced to the persistence of an ontologically and even historically false legal epistemology.

The second basic flaw is embedded in the concept of development itself. This does not mean that status-quo is to be maintained. This does not mean that the basic needs of the bulk of the population should remain unsatisfied. This means that pervert consumerism for a small population of the world and poverty for the rest of the mankind are to be simultaneously fought out. This means that world opinion is to be mobilised for the creation of a standard setting global covenant, simultaneously providing for production norm, labour condition norm and consumption norm. Ruskin's concept of "Unto the last", Gandhi's advocacy for satisfaction of basic needs of all rather than relentless pursuit of expanding the scope of living standards; revision of the Universal Declaration of Human Rights incorporating collective rights and more emphasis on eco-ethics in ecological concern should provide the bases for a paradigm shift.

The study by exposing many faceted perversions of the system at work, will stir many to think, to act. I congratulate the authors and their research team for their factual and conceptual message.

New Delhi
April 15, 1998

B. K. Roy Burman

PREFACE

THIS study deals with the impact of the setting up of a number of irrigation, power and mining projects in the Sonbhadra district of Uttar Pradesh. The area is inhabited largely by the Scheduled Castes, including twelve communities who are tribals, basically. The area was a Partially Excluded Area, in terms of the Government of India Act 1935, till the advent of freedom, after which it lost its protected character. In these circumstances the results of industrialization, combined with lack of planning for rehabilitation, have been disastrous for the entire affected population, specially the Scheduled and Backward Castes.

The Tribal Development Division, Ministry of Welfare, Government of India which provided funds for this study deserves our grateful thanks. Sri P.K. Mohanty, Director (TD) has to be specially mentioned for his help and suggestions.

The need for such a study was mooted by Sri K. R. Rhati, then Secratary, Social Welfare, Government of Uttar Pradesh Our special thanks are due to him as his initiative made the study possible.

Dr. B.D. Sharma the last Commissioner for Scheduled Castes and Scheduled Tribes gave us the benefit of discussions and guidance. We have to thank him, and also Prof. K.N. Sharma, formerly of the I.I.T., Kanpur and Prof. B.K. Roy Burman who were consulted at the planning stages of the study. Prof. Sharma subsequently made comprehensive suggestions for recasting the report in its present form and Prof. Roy Burman graciously agreed to write its Foreword.

In the context of two National Thermal Power Corporation projects in Sonbhadra district, the World Bank assumes a position of importance. We had, therefore, approached Dr. Michael M. Cernea, Senior Adviser, Sociology and Social Policy of the Bank for his writings and other material relating to the rehabilitation policies of the World Bank. Dr. Cernea not only promptly provided all the material but also evinced keen interest in our work for which we are obliged to him.

The Ethnographic and Folk Culture Society—with which we have been associated for several decades and for which we have a special attachment as it was founded by our great teacher of anthropology, the late Prof. D.N. Majumdar—extended the infrastructural facilities required for the work. For this we have to express our gratitude to the Society's General Secretary, Dr. B.R.K. Shukla and its Hony. Treasurer, Sri J.N. Shukla at that time. The latter was extremely helpful in the project's financial management.

We would be failing in our duty if we do not mention the valuable help that was received from several Life Members of the Society. Sri Sukant K. Chaudhury, Lecturer, Department of Sociology, Lucknow University, has to be mentioned specially for commenting on the draft chapters. Sri Tarun Khanna helped in collecting some primary and secondary data and Sri P.K. Tewari, Department of Anthropology, J.N. Degree College, Lucknow, provided several rare books.

The institutional help received in the field came from several sources. It would be difficult to recount it all. However, the General Manager and officers of the Singrauli Super Thermal Power Project, Shaktinagar and the Northern Coalfields Ltd., Singrauli, are to be remembered with warmth. In the NTPC headquarters, Sri Mata Prasad then Executive Director, took keen interest in our work and helped in various ways. Several district officers and senior officers of the Government of U.P., at Lucknow, particularly the Board of Revenue, State Electricity Board and Secretariat Departments gave us the benefit of their knowledge and discussions and we thank them all.

The late Sri Prem Bhai of the Banwasi Seva Ashram, Govindpur, was an institution by himself in this area. Being an old friend he ungrudgingly provided us with important basic data, and a perspective through long discussions. Sri Avadhesh of the M.P. Lokayan Lokhit Samiti, Singrauli also helped similarly. The Mirzapur branch of the Servants of India Society generously played host as our field centre for which our sincere thanks are due to Sri A.N. Misra its Life Member and Sri Leeladhar Yadav, Principal of the Birla Vidya Mandir, Muirpur. Sri Amit and Alka Sahai helped in modifying the map from the Mirzapur Census Hand Book—1971, used in this book.

The study would have never taken shape without the hard work and long hours put in by our research team and the stenographer. Our publisher Sri M.C. Mittal of the Inter-India Publications, New Delhi can never be thanked enough for his interest in this book at different stages.

Lastly, we have to heartily thank Smt. Manorama Saksena, wife of the first author, for the ungrudging help and warm hospitality extended to all of us at different stages of our work.

Lucknow
July 31, 1998

H.S. Saksena
Chandra Sen

CONTENTS

CONTENTS

LIST OF TABLES

Page

List of Map

1

INTRODUCTION

ONE of the chief characteristics of tribal communities is eco-geographic by nature, i.e. the nature of habitation, which is usually a forest or hilly area. The relationship between a community and its area of habitation leads to a whole range of social, economic and ritual configurations which is so delicately balanced that the community can hardly conceive a break from its hoary moorings. Even the tribal communities which are migratory in character or those who follow a ritualistic belief in changing the sites of their villages/houses after an incidence of death, epidemic, etc., follow a well-defined pattern of movement within a specified area. Such a bond between the tribal and his milieu strongly discourages mobility even among the individuals. Till the 40s of the current century there were hardly any factors which would cause a disturbance in this relationship as there was negligible industrial and related activity in the tribal heartlands. A deliberate state policy of *laissez faire* left the tribal communities in isolation and undisturbed in their own areas.

The country's era of planned development was initiated in the early 50s. The main objective of the plans was a movement towards higher productivity and greater equality. Since then the country has witnessed great leaps in power production and irrigation through multi-purpose power and irrigation projects and dams along with extensive mining for coal and iron, giant steel mills and a host of other infrastructural and productive activities. These were sinews of sustained economic growth aimed at meeting recurring power shortage as also for building a sound industrial base for the country.

The focii of all such developmental efforts are mostly the resource-rich regions, many of which are in the hilly and forested areas, inhabited by the tribals. The displacements caused by this leap of the country towards the twenty-first century have been enormous. "India is currently a developing country with the largest dam construction programme and correspondingly with the most massive involuntary dislocation" (Cernea 1991).

The scenario of impact of all such projects is characterised by several aspects, viz. the lack of comprehensive data about the quantum of displacement and the resultant rehabilitation effort; number of persons belonging to the Scheduled Tribes and Scheduled Castes forming a part of the Project Affected Persons (PAPs) which is about 40 per cent (India 1985: 18-19); and the dismal state of rehabilitation with few efforts at its evaluation and resultant corrections.

Fernandes (1989, 1997) examines the situation of displacement and rehabilitation during the last four decades (1951-1990) on an all-India basis. Categorising the projects responsible for displacement into mineral resources projects, irrigation and hydel dam projects, industries, national parks, wild life sanctuaries and others (roads, airports, railways, etc.), he has examined the extent of rehabilitation; and has taken into consideration separately the tribal areas and the tribals. The picture that emerges is rather alarming (Table 1.1).

It is obvious that the problem of the Project Affected Persons is enormous as the statistics from Table 1.1, which can hardly be taken as final, show. Only 25 per cent of the PAPs have been rehabilitated, the quality and

TABLE 1.1 : **Displacement and Rehabilitation due to Various Projects in India**

('000 Persons)

Sr. No.	Types	Numbers Displaced			Numbers Rehabilitated		Backlog	
		Total	Tribal region	Tribal	Total	Tribal (based on % in Tribal region)	Total	Tribal
1	2	3	4	5	6	7	8	9
1.	Mines	2,100	1,415	1,200	525	300	1,575	900
2.	Dams	14,000	7,000	5,300	3,500	1,315	10,500	3,945
3.	Industries	1,300	300	260	325	65	950	195
4.	Wild life	600	600	500	150	125	562	375
5.	Others	500	200	150	125	40	375	110
	Total	18,500	9,515	7,410	4,625	1,850	13,962	5,560
	Percentage			40	25	40	75	40.07

durability of which may vary a great deal.

In the context of this poor state of rehabilitation, the present study carried out in 1992-93 aims at understanding the empirical situation of the oustees of various projects in the Sonbhadra district of Uttar Pradesh. In this area people have faced even multiple displacements which mainly started in the year 1960 with the construction of the Rihand dam and reservoir and has been a continuous process. Thus, the study tries to bring out the travails and tribulations faced by the people of the area in the past three decades.

Industrialisation and Displacement in Sonbhadra

The district comprises of two tahsils : Dudhi in the southern part and Robertsganj in the northern part. A part of Robertsganj tahsil and the entire Dudhi tahsil lie south of the Kaimur hill range. The tribal and Scheduled Caste population of the district live mostly in this area, excepting the Kol who reside in several blocks lying both north and south of the Kaimur range. As such industrialisation in the portion lying south of Kaimur as well as in the rest of the district has affected the tribal population.

Among the initial projects in the area, the Cement factories at Churk and Dala and the Ahraura Dam located north of the Kaimur range caused displacement of some Kol families, besides others. The cement factories were set up during the First Five Year Plan and expanded in two subsequent plans. The two factories have undergone a modernisation programme at a sizeable cost in the early 80s. The Ahraura Dam is a medium irrigation project started in the First Plan and completed in the Second Plan with a irrigation potential of 8870 ha. Compared to the southern part of the district these activities were quite modest.

In the south of the Kaimur range the first major project, the Rihand Dam, was started in 1948 but the work was suspended in 1949. It was restarted in 1955 and completed during the Third Plan. The dam produces hydro-electricity. Next came the Obra hydel power project of the Uttar Pradesh Electricity Board (UPSEB), 32 kms. down stream of Rihand Dam, started in the Second Plan and completed during the Third Plan. Subsequently, its expansion was taken up in the Fourth and the Fifth Five Year Plans. The Anpara Thermal Power Project of the UPSEB was started in 1979 on the left bank of Rihand Reservoir. It is still under construction. The National Thermal Power Corporation (NTPC) started its Singrauli Super Thermal Project at Shaktinagar in October 1977 and its further expansion was undertaken in the 80s and completed in early 90s. NTPC's second thermal power project came up at Bijpur (Rihand Nagar) on the North-eastern side of the Rihand Reservoir. The Project was started in the year 1982 and is presently undergoing expansion. The Northern Coalfields Limited (NCL) started the exploitation of coal bearing areas contiguously located in U.P. and M.P. in the year 1975. Three of their seven coalfields are located in U.P. Besides, there is only one irrigation project (Kanhar) located in the Dudhi tahsil. This project was started in 1974-75 to create an irrigation potential of 32,000 ha. It is being constructed at a rather slow pace due to shortage of funds. The target was to complete it during the Eighth Plan which is not likely to be achieved.

In the private sector, the Birlas set up the Hindustan Aluminium Co. (HINDALCO) at Renukoot near Pipri during the Second Plan followed by the Kanoria's Chemical Plant in the same vicinity. Recently in 1986 Birlas have added a Hytech Carbon Plant at some distance from HINDALCO.

There is a great deal of confusion regarding the actual number of persons/families displaced by the above mentioned projects. Even to begin with there is no reliable data regarding PAPs from the Rihand Dam built in 1961 as the people—mostly tribals and Backward and Scheduled Castes—were asked by the authorities to move and settle in the neighbouring forest area. A substantial number of these persons reportedly moved to M.P. (Sarguja district) and towards Babhni (eastern Sonbhadra district) where they had tribal and kinship ties. Nothing much is known about their numbers and post-displacement conditions. Then, in so far as all the subsequent displacements are concerned only the actual owners of agricultural lands or houses were compensated in cash and thereby reckoned. As per the provisions of the Land Acquisition Act, 1894 (LAA) no compensation was due to the landless persons, agricultural labourers, artisans, etc. whose population was substantial and this renders all records of displaced persons incomplete.

According to a recent estimate the displaced families add up to at least 36,000 (Table 1.2).

TABLE 1.2 : **Project-wise break up of Displaced Families in Sonbhadra (Estimated)**

Sl. No.	Name of the Project	Number of Families displaced
1.	Rihand Dam	10,000
2.	Cement Factories	800
3.	Kanhar Irrigation Project	2,000
4.	Singrauli area	
	(a) NTPC (b) NCL	5,000
5.	UPSEB	
	(a) Anpara (b) Obra	1,500
6.	World Food Programme Forestry Project	1,000
7.	NTPC Bijpur	700
8.	Roads, Railways, Airstrips, High-tension lines, etc.	15,000
	Total	36,000

Source : Banawasi Seva Ashram, Govindpur, Sonbhadra

Out of these, about 10,000 families of Rihand oustees have faced multiple displacement in the past—"4 or 5 displacements—the record is 6 displacements in 25 years" (EDF 1990).

Research Design

The incidence of displacement in this comparatively small and remote district of Uttar Pradesh—having an area of only 6,788 sq. km. and a population of 10,75,041 in 1991—has been tremendous on the people, the environment and the economy. The pace of industrialisation which started nearly three decades ago has been picking up specially after the substantial extension of their coalfields by the NCL and the NTPC making it the 'power capital' of India. However, during these three decades of industrialisation no comprehensive picture of the actual situation in the field and conditions of the affected people were put forth through any study or official report. Only a couple of voluntary agencies, such as Lokayan and Lokhit Samiti, Singrauli and the Banwasi Seva Ashram, Govindpur, were agitating, discussing and disseminating information about the situation.

B.D. Sharma as Commissioner for Scheduled Castes and Scheduled Tribes took active interest in the problems which were multiplying fast and extensively in the area. In his twenty-eighth report he commented bitterly on the "processes of deprivation which are being accentuated by the forces of development" and described how "on the outskirts of Shaktinagar in Mirzapur District (Uttar Pradesh) the administration, backed by the P.A.C., (Provincial Armed Constabulary) was warning the people with the blare of a mike, at the dead of night, in the midst of monsoon season, to move out to a new site where some make-shift sheds had been put up and a few tents pitched, for the people to be huddled into, little realising that during this season even birds do not move out and the mendicants also pause for *Chaturmass*". (Commissioner 1988 : 12).

In his next report he gave a more focussed attention to the situation created by such displacements throughout the country treating Sonbhadra as a case study. He pointed out the failure of the administration and the project authorities to protect the legitimate interests of the tribals and Scheduled Castes particularly on the following counts :

(i) Due to the absence or incompleteness of record of rights tribal lands were grabbed by outsiders. It is a *loot* which is going on in the Sonbhadra . . . There is no count of big farmers and also big projects which have been established in the area after independence. Nobody has bothered . . . Government and the administration are blissfully engrossed in developmental work.

(ii) People displaced by Rihand dam were moved and asked to occupy and cultivate forest lands but received no *pattas* and even forty years after these people left their original houses they have no place which they can call their own. Subsequently, many were displaced more than once due to other projects.

(iii) On displacement, promises were made and not fulfilled–Nehru promised them electricity from Rihand dam, which has not so far been given to them though it is reaching out to distant corners of the country.

(iv) The right of the displaced persons has remained circumscribed only to cash compensation. Whatever was given, besides the compensation, was by way of concession only. That is why the Central Government had recently withdrawn its circular on employment which had advised all industrial establishments to provide a job to one member of each displaced family.

(Commissioner 1990 : 253-54)

placements were faced and the resultant conditions of the peoples, we collected a large number of 'focussed autobiographies' from both the community leaders and ordinary individuals. This material has been presented here selectively.

(v) In the last stage we had discussions with the officers concerned in the different projects whenever they were willing to freely discuss their policy and its implementation largely basing our interviews on the material collected earlier from the projects through a brief questionnaire. Interviews with prominent functionaries from the non-government organisations (NGOs) operating in the area and some other leaders were also conducted.

2

THE SETTING

THE Sonbhadra district was created in 1989 by taking out the two southern tehsils of Robertsganj and Dudhi from the Mirzapur district. It is, thus, situated south of Mirzapur district deriving its name from river Son. It is bound in the north by Mirzapur and Varanasi districts of Uttar Pradesh, in the east by Palamau and Shahabad districts of Bihar and in the south and west by the Sarguja and Sidhi districts of Madhya Pradesh. The headquarters of the district is Robertsganj, situated on the north-west side of the district (See Map).

Topography

The geographical area of Sonbhadra is 6,788 sq. kms. It is a tableland stretching from the summit of Vindhyan Scarp southwards to the Kaimur range and the valley of the Son river and beyond this lie the jungle-clad ravines and scarps with hill-enriched alluvial basins like Singrauli here and there. Drake-Brockman (1911) provides a detailed account of the area. This tract consists for the most part of numerous parallel lines of rocky hills, of no great height, but rugged and impracticable, and clothed with jungle usually of a stunted and ill-grown description. Entering it at Chopan, a traveller, whose gaze falls on the blue waters of the river, flowing swiftly over broad stretches of silver sand, with the dark castellated heights of Mangeswar forming an imposing background all along the north as far as the eye can reach, would at once be struck by the beauty of the scenery but as he went further south, the splendid vision would fade away into stretches of arid waste, intersected by ridges and *nalas*, only opening out in a few places to enclose low lying patches of culturable soil. Starting from Agori, there is first of all a long, narrow strip of fertile land, bordering on the Son and backed by some rows of hills. Crossing these at Gaeghat, where the fertile land ceases, one reaches the Kon valley. This is fairly extensive and runs parallel with the Son. After the Kon valley, with the exception of a little scattered cultivation near the Pandu river, no more culturable land is seen till the passes near Pandu Chhattan are surmounted and Jorukhar, the northern outpost of the Dudhi valley, is reached. The Dudhi valley is bounded on the north by the rugged mass of broken country which lies between it and the Son; on the east, by the Palamau district; and, on the south, by the southern range of hills, of which Gonda has the highest elevation. It is a fertile, prosperous valley, which is much wider and more extensive to the south, where it opens out around Muirpur and merges into the Singrauli basin. The Singrauli basin is triangular in shape, its base lying around Kota on the Rewa (Sidhi) frontier, and the apex running nearly up to the Audi hills. The soil is a rich alluvial loam, and cultivation is in a better state than in Dudhi owing to the absence of intersecting rivers. These three valleys together with the strip along the Son in Agori, contain practically all the land available for cultivation. The area of the whole Sonpar tract is about 1700 sq. miles but the population is very sparse and scanty, (Drake-Brockman 1911).

The main river of the district is the Son. Besides, there are four medium sized streams—Belan, Karamnar, Rihand and Kanhar and a host of minor channels. South of the Kaimur, there is only one small stream, the Ganghar which flows into the Son on its left bank but, south of the river, the Dudhi and Singrauli basins are drained by a large number of tributary channels which like the Ajhir, Bichchi, Lauwa and Thema either join the Rihand and Kanhar or like the Bijui flow into the Son.

The soil of the district is of varying type. In the plateau it is generally a stiff and sallow red clay. In the fertile strip lying at the foot of the Kaimur there are large areas of excellent loam and clay, such as obtained in the Ganges valley, as well as of a fine black soil resembling the black cotton soil of Bundelkhand and Central India. Between the plateau and the north bank of the Son, there intervenes a 10 km. stretch of light sandy alluvial soil. In the tract beyond Son the cultivation that exists depends upon the availability of stiff clays or a loose sandy soil, according to the elevation of the patches of tillage. The Singrauli basin, however, is covered with a rich black loam overlying the well-known boulder drift of the Talchir series, which comes to the surface in the higher portions of the basin. The cultivated basin of the adjoining tahsil of Dudhi is also similar in character.

Climate

The climate of the district is characterised by a hot summer, a pleasant monsoon, and a severe winter. The year may be divided into four seasons. The cold seasons from about the middle of November to the end of February is followed by the hot season from March to about June. The south-west monsoon season is from the middle of June to the end of September. October and the first-half of November constitute the post-monsoon season. The average annual rainfall in the district is 1,129.9 mm. It generally decreases from the south-east to the north-west. About 80 per cent of the annual rainfall in the district takes place during the south-west monsoon months from June to September, August being the month of the heaviest rainfall. The variation in the rainfall from

The then Secretary, Social Welfare, Uttar Pradesh took note of the comments in these reports and suggested that a research study of the situation in Sonbhadra, particularly covering the tribals and Scheduled Castes should be undertaken. We had a long standing interest in the area. Majumdar had started studies around Dudhi in 1940s and the research team for *Chhor Ka Ek Gaon* included the co-author of the present study. Both the authors had been visiting the area from time to time since 1960s. Therefore, we planned the study with all this background knowledge. The portrayal of the field situation in Sonbhadra by the Commissioner for Scheduled Castes and Scheduled Tribes (1988, 1990) indicated the main thrusts or directions for our enquiry. Obviously, the study was intended to probe extensively as well as intensively the socio-economic conditions of the PAP and explore the directions in which the rehabilitation programme should desirably be pursued. Briefly the objectives of the study were :

(i) To gauge the extent of displacements including multiple displacements and their impact on the economic bases and pattern of life of the affected populations, particularly the tribals and the Scheduled Castes;

(ii) to examine the rehabilitation measures incorporated in the projects and policies of the different agencies responsible for displacements;

(iii) to evaluate the effectiveness of the delivery of the rehabilitation measures, their adequacy and suitability;

(iv) to identify the reasons which retarded the efficacy of rehabilitation package, such as legal and policy lacunae, planning and managerial infirmities, approach of the personnel responsible for rehabilitation, etc.;

(v) to document the present economic and

community status of the affected populations and determine whether they had regained atlest their pre-displacement levels; and

(vi) to suggest further measures that need to be taken in order to make rehabilitation effective, enduring and successful.

The research design formulated to achieve the above objectives based the study mainly on primary data with a balanced mix of the use of secondary sources of data and comprised the following :

(i) Examination of the census data, government reports and materials published by the projects and non-government organisations in order to make an assessment of the dimensions of displacement and their main theatres. Since the census data was found to have only a limited utility due to heavy migration into the area and the creation of a new district other sources were found to be more useful.

(ii) Collection of field data about the PAPs at three levels—the community (caste/tribe), the family and the individuals. The base line data for the community level was obtained from three published sources namely the old gazetteer of Mirzapur district (Drake-Brockman 1911), *Chhor ka Ek Gaon* (Majumdar 1960) and the revised district gazetteer (Mishra 1988). These documents provided ethnographic material relating to the tribes and also the Scheduled Castes, spanning a period of more than 70 years and this was added to and compared with the data of 1992-93 collected from the field.

(iii) At the family level the data collection was made on a wide base. The important conglomerations of displacement or rehabilitation were identified and in six of these—which included oustees from the Rihand dam, two NTPC and one UPSEB power plants, NCL coalfields and the Kanhar dam in Dudhi tahsil—a schedule was administered among 1038 families, roughly 10 per cent of the oustee families. The families were selected randomly, with a broad stratification giving overwhelming representation to the Scheduled Castes and tribals (*adivasis*). The Backward castes were also included along with just a few other higher castes for the sake of comparison and keeping in view, Majumdar's (1960) concept of a 'fringe village', as developed for the area. The schedule was first tested and then finalised. Obviously, the focus was on the family structure, its comparative economic base and assets (before and after displacement), displacement conditions, compensations and present living conditions and the informants' assessment of losses or gains in the area of economic base, living conditions, cultural and social relations or the 'social fabric' (Cernea 1991: 194-6). The schedule contained both structured, semi-structured and open-ended questions. It also provided room for additional qualitative informations and comments. The quantitative data was processed with the help of computer and the qualitative and miscellaneous informations were analysed through standard interpretations.

The anthropological techniques of social research place a good degree of emphasis and reliance on autobiographical material (Madge 1953). Since our objective was to recapitulate the previous conditions of living, the way dis-

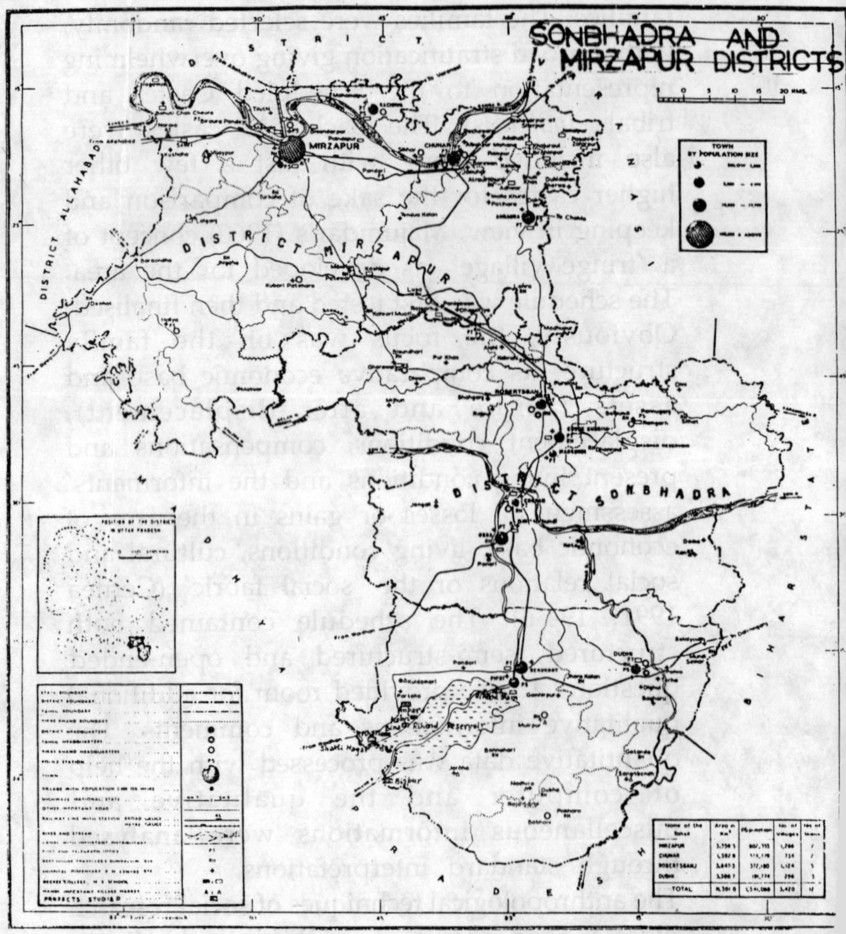

MAP 1.1 : *Sonbhadra and Mirazapur Districts*

which flows into the Son on its left bank but, south of the river, the Dudhi and Singrauli basins are drained by a large number of tributary channels which like the Ajhir, Bichchi, Lauwa and Thema either join the Rihand and Kanhar or like the Bijui flow into the Son.

The soil of the district is of varying type. In the plateau it is generally a stiff and sallow red clay. In the fertile strip lying at the foot of the Kaimur there are large areas of excellent loam and clay, such as obtained in the Ganges valley, as well as of a fine black soil resembling the black cotton soil of Bundelkhand and Central India. Between the plateau and the north bank of the Son, there intervenes a 10 km. stretch of light sandy alluvial soil. In the tract beyond Son the cultivation that exists depends upon the availability of stiff clays or a loose sandy soil, according to the elevation of the patches of tillage. The Singrauli basin, however, is covered with a rich black loam overlying the well-known boulder drift of the Talchir series, which comes to the surface in the higher portions of the basin. The cultivated basin of the adjoining tahsil of Dudhi is also similar in character.

Climate

The climate of the district is characterised by a hot summer, a pleasant monsoon, and a severe winter. The year may be divided into four seasons. The cold seasons from about the middle of November to the end of February is followed by the hot season from March to about June. The south-west monsoon season is from the middle of June to the end of September. October and the first-half of November constitute the post-monsoon season. The average annual rainfall in the district is 1,129.9 mm. It generally decreases from the south-east to the north-west. About 80 per cent of the annual rainfall in the district takes place during the south-west monsoon months from June to September, August being the month of the heaviest rainfall. The variation in the rainfall from of Mangeswar forming an imposing background all along the north as far as the eye can reach, would at once be struck by the beauty of the scenery but as he went further south, the splendid vision would fade away into stretches of arid waste, intersected by ridges and *nalas*, only opening out in a few places to enclose low lying patches of culturable soil. Starting from Agori, there is first of all a long, narrow strip of fertile land, bordering on the Son and backed by some rows of hills. Crossing these at Gaeghat, where the fertile land ceases, one reaches the Kon valley. This is fairly extensive and runs parallel with the Son. After the Kon valley, with the exception of a little scattered cultivation near the Pandu river, no more culturable land is seen till the passes near Pandu Chhattan are surmounted and Jorukhar, the northern outpost of the Dudhi valley, is reached. The Dudhi valley is bounded on the north by the rugged mass of broken country which lies between it and the Son; on the east, by the Palamau district; and, on the south, by the southern range of hills, of which Gonda has the highest elevation. It is a fertile, prosperous valley, which is much wider and more extensive to the south, where it opens out around Muirpur and merges into the Singrauli basin. The Singrauli basin is triangular in shape, its base lying around Kota on the Rewa (Sidhi) frontier, and the apex running nearly up to the Audi hills. The soil is a rich alluvial loam, and cultivation is in a better state than in Dudhi owing to the absence of intersecting rivers. These three valleys together with the strip along the Son in Agori, contain practically all the land available for cultivation. The area of the whole Sonpar tract is about 1700 sq. miles but the population is very sparse and scanty, (Drake-Brockman 1911).

The main river of the district is the Son. Besides, there are four medium sized streams—Belan, Karamnar, Rihand and Kanhar and a host of minor channels. South of the Kaimur, there is only one small stream, the Ganghar

2

THE SETTING

THE Sonbhadra district was created in 1989 by taking out the two southern tehsils of Robertsganj and Dudhi from the Mirzapur district. It is, thus, situated south of Mirzapur district deriving its name from river Son. It is bound in the north by Mirzapur and Varanasi districts of Uttar Pradesh, in the east by Palamau and Shahabad districts of Bihar and in the south and west by the Sarguja and Sidhi districts of Madhya Pradesh. The headquarters of the district is Robertsganj, situated on the north-west side of the district (See Map).

Topography

The geographical area of Sonbhadra is 6,788 sq. kms. It is a tableland stretching from the summit of Vindhyan Scarp southwards to the Kaimur range and the valley of the Son river and beyond this lie the jungle-clad ravines and scarps with hill-enriched alluvial basins like Singrauli here and there. Drake-Brockman (1911) provides a detailed account of the area. This tract consists for the most part of numerous parallel lines of rocky hills, of no great height, but rugged and impracticable, and clothed with jungle usually of a stunted and ill-grown description. Entering it at Chopan, a traveller, whose gaze falls on the blue waters of the river, flowing swiftly over broad stretches of silver sand, with the dark castellated heights placements were faced and the resultant conditions of the peoples, we collected a large number of 'focussed autobiographies' from both the community leaders and ordinary individuals. This material has been presented here selectively.

(v) In the last stage we had discussions with the officers concerned in the different projects whenever they were willing to freely discuss their policy and its implementation largely basing our interviews on the material collected earlier from the projects through a brief questionnaire. Interviews with prominent functionaries from the non-government organisations (NGOs) operating in the area and some other leaders were also conducted.

year to year is appreciable.

Geology

The district is very important from geological point of view and as such it may be divided into four tracts — the Kaimur hills, the Son valley, the hilly tract south of the Son, and the Singrauli basin. Each of these divisions has the shape of longitudinal strips stretching from east to west. The lowest, Garbandh group, usually occurs at a short distance from the Son. This group takes its name from the Garbandh table land situated close to the western boundary of Palamau and adjacent to the eastern border of Mirzapur. It consists of conglomerates, shales, carbonacious beds, limestones, porcellanites, and glauconitic sandstone. The second subdivision of the lower Vindhyans consists of trappoids and porcellanites. They are indurated, siliceous, volcanic ashes and are usually found in the immediate neighbourhood of the south bank of the Son. The third subdivision, or Kheinjua group, consists of limestones and of shale with calcareous concertions. It usually forms the northern bank of the Son and its name is derived from a range of hills lying south of the Kaimur scarp at and beyond the western boundary of the Rewa in the Son Valley. The last group in this formation is the Rohtas. It consists of thin-bedded limestones found at the foot and along the lower slopes of the Kaimur range.

Mineral Wealth

The district is rich in mineral wealth which forms a long and varied list. According to Drake-Brockman (1911), "owing to the inaccessible nature of tract, where the mineral products occur, none of them have been exploited with the exception of building stone and limestone. However, minerals like felspar, mica, epidot, limestones and marbles, corundum, lead, iron, coal, magnesite, haematite, calcite dolomite and kankar are all found in the district." Exploitation of minerals has now started and a large work force is now engaged in mining and quarrying. This work is being done by the U.P. State Mineral Development Corporation which is exploiting limestone, dolomite and some other stones, and also by private contractors. The coal deposits in the southern part of the district are being worked by the Northern Coalfields Limited, a Government of India's Undertaking.

Flora

The total area under forest is 49.1 per cent of the district. Roughly speaking about 18 per cent of the forested area of U.P. is under the reserved forests. In Sonbhadra, however there is a controversy about large areas of land notified by the Forest Department as reserved/protected forests and claimed by the cultivators, mainly tribals, as their agricultural lands because there had been no settlement and proper records of rights for most parts of the district. This matter has been discussed elsewhere in this book.

The forest vegetation of the district can be categorised as Southern/Northern Dry mixed Deciduous Forest, Dry Plants, Sal Transitional to Peninsula, Sal, Dry Deciduous Scrub, Dry Bamboo Breaks, Grass Preserves and Plantation. There is a large number of trees growing in these forests. The important ones being *Sakhu*, (Shorea robusta), *semal* (Bombax ceiba), *Aonla* (Phyllanthus embica), *Bahera* (Termainalia bellirica), *Tendu* (Diosyros melanoxylon), *Palas* or *Dhak* (Butea monosperma), *Arjun* (Terminalia arjuna), *Khair* (Acacia catechu), Bamboo, Asan (Terminalia alata), Bargad (Ficus neligeosa), *Sheesham* (Dalbergia sissoo). Among the trees the *Peepal* (Ficus bengalensis), *Aam* (Magnifera indica), *Neem* (Azadirachta indica), *Bel* (Aegle marmelos), *Jamun* (Syzyguin cuminii), *Mahuwa* (Madhuca indica), *Imli* (Tamarindus indica) and *Harr* (Terminalia chebula) are commonly grown.

The minor forest produce generally found are tendu leaves, kattha, bamboo, bagai grass, lac and gums, mahua, etc. In U.P. lac is found only in the district of Sonbhadra. However, in recent years due to the setting up of industries followed by pollution and rising population the quality of forests as well as its spread has suffered and the availability of minor forest produce has also been considerably reduced.

Fauna

The district was described as a favourite haunt of large game including tigers found occasionally. But the setting up of large scale industries, irrigation dams, mining and a network of roads has resulted in little survival of big animals. Animals like hyaena, wild dog (*Kogi*), jackals, foxes, sambhar and cheetal of deer tribe, black buck and chinkara are still found in the area.

The State of Development in the District

Sonbhadra, as stated earlier, is the southern most district of the State, contiguous to some of the backward tribal districts of Madhya Pradesh and Bihar. The headquarters of the district is situated about 300 kms. from the State capital and a direct rail link to it came only recently. Before the district was carved out even the district headquarters, Mirzapur, was in the range of 250 kms. from the southernmost part of Sonbhadra. Placing the district in a perspective of some of the indicators of development as compared to the State and the national scene (Table 2.1) and land use pattern (Table 2.2), will be of help in having an idea of the conditions in the district, industrial activities notwithstanding.

The district is overwhelmingly rural and dependent on agriculture but the cultivated area is on the lower side and the irrigation facilities are far below the State level, even though the irrigation potentials are considerable—

many rivulets and a large expanse of water reservoir (Rihand)—and the utilisation of ground water is the

TABLE 2.1 : **Some Indicators of Development**

Sl. No.	Indicators		India	U.P.	Sonbhadra
1.	Literacy (%) of population aged 7 + years	1991	52.11	41.71	26.9
2.	Population growth	1981-91	+23.50	+25.48	+38.2
3.	Density	1991	267	471	158
4.	Sex ratio	1991	929	879	862
5.	Urbanisation (%)	1991	25.7	24.8	13.4
6.	% of cultivators + Agricultural labourers to Main Workers	1991		72.2	76.9
7.	Per capita income (Rs.) 1980-81 prices	1991-92	2174	1606	NA
8.	Forest area (%)	1991	21.9	17.33	49.1
9.	Cultivated area (%)	1991	59.5	58.1	26.4
10.	Power Generation (MW)	1990	222450	18887	3000 (app.)
11.	Irrigated Area (%)	1981	31.4	61.0	26.11
12.	Power used per capita (KWH)	1991	201 (1981)	168	2.75
13.	% of villages electrified	1991	80.2 (1981)	73.9	33.8
14.	Below poverty line (%)	1987-88	29.20	33.00	NA
15.	SC population below poverty line (%)	1983-84	53.1	57.3	NA

TABLE 2.2 : **Land-Use Pattern (1991)**

('000 ha.)

Sl. No.	Land-Use	Uttar Pradesh	Sonbhadra
1.	Area sown (%)	17299 (58.1%)	180 (26.4%)
	(a) Irrigated (%)	10542 (61.0%)	47 (26.1%)
	(b) Unirrigated (%)	6799 (39.0%)	133 (73.9%)
	(c) Under double cropping (%)	8200 (47.4%)	75 (41.6%)
2.	Under Forest (%)	5162 (17.3%)	335 (49.1%)
3.	Other Uses (%)	7332 (24.5%)	167 (24.5%)
	Total area reported	29793	682

lowest (8%) among all the districts of the State. Inspite of its being the "power capital of the country", supplying a sizeable chunk of power to the northern grid, the district itself consumes very little power and the number of electrified villages is one-third only. The district population growth has been one of the largest in the State, obviously due to migrations connected with industrialisation and yet its rate of urbanisation has not kept up with this migration. The literacy rate is also low. The density of population too is very low in comparison with the State as a whole. The land use pattern indicates that almost half the area is under forests. Out of the total area sown the irrigated area is far below the state average and the area under double cropping is also comparatively low.

Some information about the district (Table 2.3) again brings out its general lack of development, specially by way of urban centres, medical and educational facilities, average length of roads, electrification, etc. In all these respects the district is substantially below the state averages indicated in parenthesis.

TABLE 2.3 : **Basic Information about Sonbhadra District**

Sl. No.	Item	Period	Description	
1.	Number of villages	1991	1346	12.6 per lac
2.	Forest Villages	1991	4	
3.	Gram Sabha	1991-92	586	
4.	Nyaya Panchayat	1991-92	66	
5.	Nagar Palika	1991-92	1	
6.	Town/Notified Area Committee	1991-92	7	
7.	Police stations			
	(a) Urban	1991-92	6	
	(b) Rural	1991-92	6	
8.	Railway stations (including halts)	1991-92	17	
9.	Post Offices			
	(a) Urban	1991-92	11	
	(b) Rural	1991-92	125	12.6 per lac (14.4)
10.	Telegraph Offices	1991-92	16	1.5 per lac
11.	Telephones	1991-92	1258	117 per lac (390)
12.	Nationalised Banks	1991-92	50	1 per 21,500
13.	Rural Banks	1991-92	10	
14.	Cooperative Banks	1991-92	10	
15.	Land Development Banks	1991-92	2	
16.	Fair Price Shops			
	(a) Urban	1991-92	89	
	(b) Rural	1991-92	427	1 per 2,100
17.	A. Education—Literacy %	1991	T 34.4	M. 47.6 F. 18.6
	B. Institutions	1991	(41.6)	(55.7) (25.3)
	(a) Junior Basic Schools	1991-92	715	66.5 per lac (57.2)
	(b) Senior Basic Shools	1991-92	96	8.9 per lac (11.2)
	(c) Higher Sec. Schools	1991-92	30	2.8 per lac (4.8)
	(d) Degree Colleges	1991-92	2	0.2 per lac (0.3)
	(e) Industrial Training Institute		1	0.1 per lac

(Contd.)

TABLE 2.3 : ***Contd.***

Sl. No.	Item	Period	Description	
18.	Medical Facilities			
	(a) Allopathic	1991-92	17	1.5 per lac (3.7)
	(b) Ayurvedic	1991-92	16	1.4 per lac (1.6)
	(c) Homeopathic	1991-92	20	1.8 per lac (0.8)
	(d) Unani	1991-92	1	0.09 per lac
19.	Family & Maternity Welfare Centre	1991-92	157	1 per 6847 persons
20.	Primary Health Centres	1991-92	29	
21.	Electrified Villages	1991-92	455	
22.	Electrified Harijan Bastis	1991-92	329	
23.	Roads per 1000 sq. km.	1990-91	117.2 (295)	km.
24.	Railway line per 1000 sq. km.	1990-91	15.2	km.

Industrialisation of the Area

The district presents a picture of contrast—on the one hand the people are backward agriculturists depending largely on unirrigated land and supplementing their income from forests and labour and on the other hand there are large areas humming with a variety of heavy projects and ancillary industrial units. Tables 2.4 and 2.5 provide a picture of heavy and medium industries in the district. New units and expansions of the existing ones are also being planned in the area contiguous to the existing ones. In fact the larger Singrauli area development plans envisage a zone of intense industrial activity including the creation of the country's power capital with a population of 10 lacs. The Madhya Pradesh and Uttar Pradesh Town Planning Organisations have been working on such a scenario. The small scale industrial units are however

TABLE 2.4 : **List of Major Industrial Units in Sonbhadra**

Sl. No.	Industries	Name of Unit & Address	Total Cost (in Rs.crores)	Persons employed	Production capacity	Production Actual
1.	Coal	M/s Singrauli Coal Field, Kakri	50.00	1000	2.5 M.T.	1.5 M.T.
2.	Coal	M/s Bina Coal Project, Bina	26.00	880	2.0 M.T.	2.0 M.T.
3.	Cement	M/s U.P. Cement Factory, Churk	30.00	1473	3.0 Lakh Tonnes	2.0 Lakh Tonnes
4.	Cement	M/s U.P. Cement Factory, Dala	13.00	1888	2.12 Lakh Tonnes	2.0 Lakh Tonnes
5.	Thermal Power	M/s Singrauli Super Thermal Power Project, Shaktinagar	1118.25	2500	2000 Mega Watts	1000 Mega Watts
6.	Thermal Power	M/s Obra Thermal Power Station, Obra	25.00	321	279 Mega Watt.	200 Mega Watt
7.	Hydel Power	M/s Rihand Hydel Power Station, Pipri	55.00	424	860.5 Mega Watt	400 Mega Watt
8.	Carbon Black	M/s Carbon Hitech, Murdhawa	43.02	248	2000 M.T.	NA
9.	Caustic Soda	M/s Kanodia Chemical Industries, Renukoot	13.00	939	53388 M.T.	51000 M.T.
10.	Aluminium Ingot	M/s Hindustan Aluminium Corporation, Renukoot	231.00	5327	77306 M.T.	77000 M.T.
11.	Thermal Power	M/s Renusagar Power Co., Renusagar	32.00	1500	270 Mega Watt	270 Mega Watt
12.	Thermal Power	M/s Rihand Nagar Super Thermal Power Project, Bijpur			NA	
13.	Thermal Power	M/s Anpara Thermal Power Project, Anpara			420	

Source : Directory of Industrial Units in Sonbhadra-1991

spread throughout the district. Table 2.5 gives the statistical data blockwise about the units which are 913 in all. The Babhni block is the most backward in this respect while Chopan has the highest number of such units.

The Projects Under Study

As mentioned earlier, six major projects have been covered in the present study. They are—(a) Rihand Reservoir, (b) Singrauli Super Thermal Power Station, Shakti Nagar, (c) Anpara Thermal Power Project, Anpara, (d) NCL Coalfields at Kakri, Bina and Khadia, (e) Rihand Nagar Super Thermal Power Project, Bijpur and (f) Kanhar Irrigation Project, Kanhar. Out of these, the Singrauli and Rihand Nagar power projects are run by NTPC, the Irrigation Project at Kanhar is being constructed by the Irrigation Department, Government of Uttar Pradesh and the Coalfields are controlled by the NCL. In this section we will discuss the pace of execution of these projects, consequent displacements, submergence and rehabilitation as per the information provided mainly by the project authorities and in the next chapter we would deal with the situation as reflected in the primary data gathered from the field.

Rihand Reservoir

The first wave of major displacements was caused by the construction of Rihand Reservoir in 1960. This dam meant for generation of hydro-electricity marks the beginning of massive investment in industrial enterprises in Singrauli region. This region derives its distinct geocultural identity from links with the ancient tribal princely State of Singrauli. It comprises a large stretch (about 200 kms. long and 100 kms wide) of narrow valleys surrounded by Kaimur hills lying in the Sonbhadra district (U.P.) and Sidhi district (M.P.). Until barely 30 years ago, this region survived, far removed from modern communications and industry, on a subsistence economy of grazing, forest

TABLE 2.5 : Blockwise Details of Small Scale Industries in the District

Sr. No.	Type of Industries	Block									
		Roberts Ganj City	Roberts Ganj Rural	Cho-pan	Ghora-wal	Nagua	Chatra	Muir-pur	Dudhi	Babhni	Total
1	2	3	4	5	6	7	8	9	10	11	12
1.	Food Products	24	05	22	04	03	08	09	09	01	85
2.	Textile Products	03	—	—	—	01	03	—	05	—	12
3.	Wood & Wood Products	13	03	11	01	—	01	11	13	—	53
4.	Leather & Leather Products	02	—	—	—	—	—	01	01	—	04
5.	Paper & Paper Products	04	—	04	—	—	—	09	02	—	19
6.	Rubber, Plastic Petroleum, Coal	06	—	06	—	—	—	01	01	—	14
7.	Minerals (Non-metals)	—	—	61	—	—	—	—	—	—	61
8.	Chemicals	02	06	07	—	—	—	01	—	—	16
9.	Basic Metal & Alloy	24	02	19	—	—	—	20	10	—	75
10.	Machinery & Tools	69	05	58	—	01	02	34	06	—	175
11.	Elec. Machinery	21	—	14	01	01	01	08	02	01	49
12.	Others	19	86	11	127	19	28	37	23	—	350
	Total	187	107	213	133	25	43	131	72	02	913

Source : Directory of Industrial Units in Sonbhadra-1991

pro-duce, shifting cultivation and patches of settled cultivation.

The Rihand reservoir submerged 106 villages of Sonbhadra district and 56 villages of Sidhi district. The estimates for the persons displaced by the reservoir and dam differ and no reliable records are available. The reports of the Irrigation Department say that 9,500 families (80,000 persons) received plots on the eastern shore of the lake between Muirpur and Babhani and 40,000 persons resettled on their own between Anpara and Kota. At least 60,000 persons moved to different areas in M.P., mostly Sarguja. Another 30,000 disappeared from the region and probably scattered throughout the area (EDF 1990). At that time the Government of U.P. decided to provide between three and ten bighas of land per family which was available in the nearby areas and also some subsidy to clear the *khoont* (roots of trees). Therefore, the people moved more or less on their own and occupied lands in villages on the eastern fringe between Babhni and Bijpur and also on the south-western fringe near and between Kota-Anpara area and Singrauli. They had to occupy some of the least fertile lands like hill-slopes and rocky beds. However, with some help from the government and their own hard work, they were able to reclaim the lands and achieve a level of production which was by and large found to be satisfactory by the people concerned.

The construction of the Rihand Dam opened the area for massive industrialisation and a network of metalled roads connecting important centres of industrialisation came up within a decade. Soon after the construction of Rihand Dam, the Hindustan Aluminium Company (HINDALCO) and Kanodia Chemicals Ltd. were established. These private companies were given 10.60 sq. km. land, mostly forest areas. It is, however, likely that some 200 families were indirectly uprooted during 1963-65 as a consequence of establishment of these industries.

Singrauli Super Thermal Power Station, Shaktinagar

This project was set up in 1976 and completed in 1982. It acquired 4,350 acres of land affecting 15 villages. The details of acreage and the number of families affected can be seen from Table 2.6.

TABLE 2.6 : **Village-wise List of Area Submerged and Families Affected by Singrauli Project**

Sl. No.	Name of the Village	Year affected	Area of the village (Acre)	Number of families affected
1.	Kota	1977	692.787	192
2.	Ranibari	1977	130.445	56
3.	Barwa Bhatwari	1977	11.750	4
4.	Chilkadand	1978	1924.003	230
5.	Paraswar Chaubey	1981	51.527	39
6.	Paraswar Raja	1981	71.357	86
7.	Paraswar Babu	1981	3.805	3
8.	Khadia	1981	118.031	83
9.	Murrak	1981	87.528	75
10.	Jogichaura	1981	33.982	14
11.	Bhairwa	1981	16.064	18
12.	Mishra	1981	34.510	59
13.	Kahraul	1981	18.534	5
14.	Kahraulia	1981	9.506	21
15.	Gharsadi	1981	9.473	2
16.	Pantsagar	1981	1436.617	Non Revenue village
	Total		4349.919	887

The process of displacement took place in two stages. In the year 1977, 392 families were displaced in Chilkadand and 244 families in Paraswar Raja in 1981. The same number of displaced families were rehabilitated in village Chilkadand as well as in Paraswar Raja. In addition, 55 families were rehabilitated in Jawaharnagar. The total number of rehabilitated families comes to 691, whereas the total number of displaced families is 887. Thus the rehabilitation status of the remaining 196 families is not reflected in the information provided by the project authorities.

Cash compensation was given for agricultural land and a plot was allotted to those whose houses were acquired by the project. However, the amount of compensation and rate per acre and size of plot (house site) have not been indicated. Persons who were provided employment in the project was 370 and 24 shops were allotted amongst displaced families. Under self-employment training, a programme in carpet weaving 'is being finalised.' One labour cooperative of land oustees has been formed for doing contract jobs. It employs about 200 persons. In addition one milk distribution booth has also been allotted to labour cooperative and one PCO shop (Phone) has been allotted to a physically handicapped displaced person to whom financial assistance has also been provided.

Anpara Thermal Power Project

This project was set up in 1978 and its expansion programme is still going on. It has acquired 21.156 sq. km. of land affecting 20 villages, the important ones being Anpara, Audi, Dibulganj, Bansi, Kakri, Pipri and Balwadah. The project had displaced 1,307 families from these villages (Table 2.7).

Under rehabilitation programme developed plots of the size 60′ □ 40′ have been given to the rehabilitated families. Out of 1307 displaced families 931 families have been rehabilitated in five villages (Table 2.8).

The work in the Anpara project is going on and about 400 families are likely to be displaced soon. An amount of Rs. 2,42,50,083 was given as compensation in cash besides providing house sites as stated above. Land for land has not been given. Only 261 persons have beenprovided

TABLE 2.7 : **Village-wise Number of Families Displaced by Anpara Project**

Sl. No.	Village	Number of Families displaced
1.	Anpara	226
2.	Audi	134
3.	Dibulganj	528
4.	Bansi	4
5.	Kakri	8
6.	Pipri	133
7.	Balwadeh	247
	Total	1307

TABLE 2.8 : **Village-wise Rehabilitation of Families by Anpara Project**

Sl. No.	Name of the Village	Number of Families Rehabilitated
1.	Dibulganj	528
2.	Anpara	238
3.	Audi	145
4.	Bansi	12
5.	Kakri	8
	Total	931

employment in the project. Some persons engaged themselves with different private agencies working in the project on daily wages. In the rehabilitation areas roads, drains, drinking water facilities (through open wells, handpumps, tanks and pipe lines) playgrounds, schools, hospitals, religious places, and electricity are made available.

Northern Coalfields Limited

It has its headquarters at Singrauli in M.P. There are three coal mining projects in the Sonbhadra district, viz. Kharia, Kakri and Bina, the details of which are as follows :

(1) Kharia

This project was set up in 1981 and it will be completed in 1996. It covers an area of 15.48 sq. kms. and partly affected two villages, viz. Khadia and Chilkadand. In these villages a total tenancy area of 329 ha. (63 ha. belonging to the Scheduled Castes and 266 ha. of others) was affected and 218 families (166 Scheduled Castes and 52 others) were displaced. Each displaced family was provided with a house site of 60′ □ 40′ as per guidelines of the Government of India issued in 1984-85. Preference in employment is given to the land oustees depending upon the requirement of the project. NCL has so far offered employment to the affected persons with land holding 0.50 acres or more for general and 0.02 acres or more for the Scheduled Castes. The sum of Rs. 145.82 lakhs (out of which Rs. 28.45 lakhs went to the Scheduled Castes) was given as compensation. Land for land was not given to any one, and 269 persons (86 Scheduled Castes) got employment in the project. In order to provide house plots of size 60′ □ 40′, two rehabilitation complexes at Jawaharnagar and Ambedkarnagar were established. Civic amenities like road, drinking water facilities, street lighting, shopping centres, and schools have also been provided in these new rehabilitation colonies. The project has arranged for light vehicle driving training to 25 displaced persons. A 'shifting grant' of Rs. 1000 per family was also provided by the project.

(2) Kakri

This project was set up in 1980 and will be completed in 1993. It covers in area of 8.28 sq. kms. and has affected six villages, viz., Rehta and Kakri fully; and Bansi, Parsi, Nakri and Audhi partly. A tenancy area of 359 ha. (218 ha. of the Scheduled Castes and 141 ha. of others) of these villages was acquired by the project. Scheduled Caste families numbering 120 and 50 families of the general category were displaced from four villages, viz. Bansi, Kakri, Parsi and Rehta. NCL has provided a plot of 60′ × 40′ to each displaced family. Preference in employ-ment is provided to the land oustees depending upon the requirements of the project. The criterian adopted by NCL is to provide employment to the project affected persons with land holdings of 0.50 acre or more for others and 0.02 acre or more for the Scheduled Castes and Scheduled Tribes. Cash compensation amounting to Rs. 124.38 lakhs was paid. Out of this, Rs. 75.71 lakhs went to the Scheduled Caste PAPs. Out of 405 persons provided employment in the project, 245 were Scheduled Caste. A rehabilitation complex at Rehta has been created by NCL in which 170 families (120 others and 50 Scheduled Castes) were provided plots of the size of 60′ × 40′ free of cost. Other civic amenities like road, drinking water facilities, shopping centre, health centre, street lighting have also been provided. A sum of Rs. 1000 was also given to each family as 'shifting' grant.

(3) Bina

This project was set up in 1975 and completed in 1988. Covering as area of 12.84 sq. kms., it has affected 7 villages from which a tenancy area of 499 ha. (324 ha. from others and 125 ha. from the Scheduled Castes) was acquired. The affected villages are : (1) Jamshila, (2) Kakri, (3) Bansi, (4) Mishra, (5) Gharsani, (6) Chanduwar and (7) Barwani. Jamshila was affected fully and the rest were affected partly. However only 13 Scheduled Castes families of Bansi village were displaced each of which have been provided a house site of 60′ × 40′. A total amount of Rs. 46.31 lakhs out of which Rs. 13.00 lakhs went to Scheduled Caste families has been given as compensation in cash and 250 persons out of whom 72 are Scheduled Castes have been provided employment in the project. A sum of Rs. 1000 per family was paid to the displaced families as shifting grant.

Rihandnagar Super Thermal Power Project Bijpur

The management of this project denied us the information with regard to displacement and rehabilitation, hence this note is based on the information gathered from other sources. Bijpur is situated on the eastern flank of the Rihand reservoir at a distance of about 80 kms from Renukoot. The place gained importance after the setting up of a Super Thermal Power Project by NTPC in 1980, otherwise the periphery of the Rihand lake was dotted with medium and small sized villages. Now Bijpur is well connected with a metalled road on which regular buses ply from Renukoot, Varanasi and Mirzapur. It is not connected by a railhead so far. A motor boat service connecting Bijpur to Shaktinagar also functions. One has to travel by road via Murdhawa, Muirpur, Babhni to reach Bijpur.

Construction and development activities started in 1980 when the Project constructed its power house, staff quarters, marketing centre, picnic spot and office complexes. A small market has also come up about 1 km. before the project premises where small shops of general merchandise, food-grains, books, stationery, radio-repair, auto-repair, furniture and doctors are seen besides wayside stalls of tea, food and *pan*. Pucca roads connecting rehabilitation colonies have also been constructed. A police station is located on the main road. However, the area does not present a look of hectic industrial activity, unlike Shaktinagar, Bina or Anpara.

The villages in the vicinity were mostly the abode of Rihand oustees and many villages, a major portion of which had submerged in the reservoir, were still used for habitation. Besides usual agricultural land, the land on the banks also became available for cultivation when water receded and this land was very fertile. But now no such facilities exist.

TABLE 2.9 : **Village-wise Number of Families and Communities Affected by Kanhar Project**

Sl. No.	Name of Village	Number of Families affected	Community
1.	Barhora	29	Kharwar (2), Chero (12), Ahir (15)
2.	Laambi	26	Kharwar (23), Lohar (2), Bania (1)
3.	Gohra	07	Kharwar (5), Lohar (2)
4.	Randa Tola	04	Kharwar (2), Gond (1), Ahir (1)
5.	Bagharu	06	Gond (6)
6.	Kudri	36	Kharwar (11), Bhuiya (15), Ahir (9), Bania (1)
7.	Amwar	18	Chamar (11), Ahir (6), Gosain (1)
8.	Sundri	288	Muslim (89), Kharwar (75), Bhuiya (24), Harijan (19), Bania (28), Gond (2) Parhaiya (3), Teli (43)
9.	Suguamau	111	Bhuiya (59), Ahir (44), Baiga (6), Bania (2)
10.	Bheeshu	176	Kharwar (68), Baiga (13), Lohar (1), Ahir (94)
11.	Korchi	163	Kharwar (58), Harijan (20), Kumhar (2), Muslim (1) Bania (7), Bhuiya (73)
	Total	864	

Kanhar Irrigation Project

This large irrigation project was launched in 1978 at an estimated cost of Rs. 55.80 crores. An earth dam (3.24 kms. long and 39.90 metres high) on river Kanhar and a canal system for irrigation was to be constructed. The length of the main canal and its subsidiaries being 141.45 kms. and 150 kms. respectively, with an annual irrigation potential of 81,828 acres of land in Dudhi and Robertsganj tahsils of Sonbhadra district and some parts of the adjoining Bihar State.

The project has not been completed so far while its cost has also gone up to Rs. 122.49 crores. The residential staff quarters of the project have been constructed in Dudhi, Dhanaura, Rajkhar and at the dam site but work on the irrigation system has not been started owing to the delay in completion of the dam itself. The basic information we had asked from the project authorities was obtained informally from their office. Land from the cultivators of 11 villages was acquired by the Project at the rate of Rs. 4500 per bigha for dam, canal and residential quarters. The details relating to the dispalcements are at Table 2.9

A word about the area and its comparison with other projects for power, coalfields, etc. is important. The Kanhar Irrigation Dam is located about 26 kms. from Dudhi Tahsil headquarters and is about 100-125 kms. away from the Rihand reservoir around which the power projects and coalfields which caused multiple displacements of the local population have been setup. Though this Project was taken up in 1978 yet it has not been completed even to this day causing a lot of problems to the people of the area whose lands have been acquired but irrigation facilities have not been provided. However, a good number of families whose land has been acquired and who have also received the compensation are still cultivating their lands, growing whatever is possible. Some families have left their original home because they had no means of livelihood. The Project authorities have not provided any rehabilitation facilities like house-sites or set up rehabilitation colonies so far. An official of the Project informed us that the displaced families were initially offered house sites at Bagharu village but they did not agree to it. In a way the problem of displacement and rehabilitation in this area is not acute and thus a contrast to power projects or coalfields.

3

THE PEOPLE AND THEIR CULTURE

THE fact that Sonbhadra was a part of the Mirzapur district till 1989 causes certain difficulties in presenting and analysing the census and gazetteers' data. Therefore, in this section we have used the data relating to Sonbhadra wherever it was separately available but at places the data for the Mirzapur district had to be used.

According to 1981 census, the Mirzapur district had a Hindu population of 94.28 per cent while the Muslim population was 5.42 per cent and other religious groups, viz. Christian, Bauddha, Jain and others constituted 0.30 per cent of the population.

The Hindus included representatives of no fewer than 75 separate castes, excluding their sub-divisions. The district presented a greater variety in the composition of its population than did other districts of the State. Most of the castes were however, those which were to be found in other parts of the State as well. There were the Brahmin, Rajput and Bania among the higher castes. Then there were a number of intermediary castes — Ahir, Kurmi, Kewat, Teli, Lohar, Gaderia, Koiri, Kahar, Nai, Lunia and Mallah mostly included in the list of the Backward Castes issued by the Government of U.P. This picture is also valid, generally, for the area which now forms Sonbhadra district.

In the undivided district the Scheduled Caste population was constituted by two main categories. In the first category were those Scheduled Castes which were, by and large, found all over the State and in Sonbhadra district as well, such as the Chamar, Dhobi, Basor, Dom, etc. In this category the Chamar were the most nu-merous. The second category included the 'tribals' listed as Scheduled Castes residing almost exclusively in Sonbhadra district or in the adjoining districts also, such as the Kol.

The Muslims were mostly constituted by the Sheikh and several occupational groups such as the Julaha, Behana, Darzi, Nai and Faqir all included in the State list of Muslim Backward Castes.

Some basic data relating to the people of the district such as the growth of population, sex ratio, population density, rural-urban ratio, literacy and the ratio of workers to non-workers has been given in Table 2.1. We may, therefore, now examine the economic structure of the population. According to the 1991 census (Table 3.1) The work-force consisted of 4,10,636 persons (3,05,381 males and 1,05,255 females) and they were 38.23 per cent of the total population. Significantly, female workers were 34.43 per cent of the total main workers in the district, as compared to 11.73 per cent for the State. The occupational structure of the main workers indicates that 76.9 per cent of them were engaged directly in agriculture (agriculturist and agricultural labour) as compared to the percentage of 53.27 per cent for the State. The percentage of those engaged in manufacturing/processing (household and non-household) was, however, substantially higher—7.1 per cent, as compared to 2.4 for Uttar Pradesh as a whole. The percentage of main workers engaged in other services (8.2%) also compared well with the State percentage of 9.98. Blockwise, the projects studied by us are located mostly in the Muirpur block followed by the Babhani and

TABLE 3.1 : **Block-wise Occupational Structure of the Population in Sonbhadra District—1991**

Sl. No.	Category	Block/Number								Percentage	
		Ghora-wal	Roberts-ganj	Chatra	Nagwa	Chopan	Muir-pur	Dudhi	Babhani	District	State
1.	Agriculturist	35066	23063	14809	14756	34706	31089	23673	16409	47.4	53.27
2.	Agri. labour	25496	25325	13748	10624	18447	10938	10899	4797	29.5	18.94
3.	Livestock, forestry, fishing and hunting	303	436	125	95	292	418	495	111	0.8	0.72
4.	Mining/quarrying	73	88	4	2	219	3942	59	4	1.1	0.08
5.	Manufacturing, processing and repair in other than household sector	1798	977	271	210	483	769	410	43	1.3	2.41
6.	Manufacturing, processing and repairs in household sector	2609	1267	305	212	3241	1656	502	81	5.8	5.34
7.	Construction	132	384	59	29	254	3683	340	23	1.4	1.24
8.	Trade and commerce	730	904	357	182	702	2747	659	133	3.2	6.17
9.	Transport/storage and communication	216	708	92	28	283	1053	198	30	1.2	1.86
10.	Other services	1191	1982	737	226	1211	13341	967	333	8.2	9.98

Dudhi blocks. In Muirpur the percentage of non-agriculture based workers is the highest (38.5%), followed by Chopan, Robertsganj and Dudhi. Non-workers numbered 6,24,148 (2,68,718 males and 3,55,430 females).

The 1991 census data relating to individual Scheduled Castes has not become available so far except for their total population and sex-wise and rural-urban breakup (Table 3.2).

TABLE 3.2 : **Population of Scheduled Castes — 1991**

Sl. No.	Population	Rural	Urban	Total
1.	Population			
	(a) Male	231106	9849	240955
	(b) Female	208582	7335	215917
	(c) Total	439688	17184	456872
2.	% of District	47.3	11.8	42.5
3.	Sex ratio	905	700	896
4.	Growth Rate (1981-91)	NA	NA	+ 33.3%

Scheduled Caste-wise population in Mirzapur district according to the 1981 census (Table 3.3) indicates that the Agaria, Baheliya, Baiga, Baiswar, Balmiki, Bhuiya, Chamar, Chero, Dhangar, Dharkar, Dhobi, Dom, Dusadh, Ghasia, Gond, Hela, Kharwar, Khatik, Kol, Kori, Korwa, Majhwar, Musahar, Nat, Pankha, Parahiya, Pasi and Patari were numerically the largest Scheduled Castes. The other Scheduled Castes (34 in number) were either not found or found in negligible numbers, i.e. less than 500. The area now comprising Sonbhadra too is having a similar Scheduled Caste-wise composition. Of these the Agaria, Baiga, Baiswar, Bhuiya, Chero, Gond, Kharwar, Kol and Majhwar have tribal origins. Besides, minor tribal groups are the Korwa, Parahiya and Patari. Chamar, Dhobi, Dusadh, Hela, Khatik, Kori and Pasi are

TABLE 3.3 : **Profile of Major Scheduled Castes in Mirzapur District—1981**

Sl. No.	Name of Caste		Population	Main workers	Cultivators	Agricultural labourers	Livestock	Mining and Quarrying	Household industries	Other than House hold industries	Construction	Trade and Commerce	Stores and transport	Other services	Marginal workers
1	2		3	4	5	6	7	8	9	10	11	12	13	14	15
1.	Agaria :	T	6530	2913	1355	1420	727	—	42	29	3	5	—	22	13
		R	6486	2899	1354	1417	638	—	42	26	3	5	—	16	13
		U	44	14	1	3	89	—	—	3	—	—	—	6	—
2.	Baiga :	T	8296	3685	1726	1871	—	—	5	4	18	14	11	31	302
		R	8212	3664	1719	1860	—	—	5	4	18	14	11	31	302
		U	84	21	7	11	—	—	—	—	—	—	—	—	—
3.	Baheliya :	T	678	244	131	49	—	—	—	—	—	—	—	—	—
		R	545	202	131	46	—	—	—	—	—	—	—	—	—
		U	133	42	—	3	—	—	—	—	—	—	—	—	—
4.	Balmiki :	T	737	296	5	2	2	—	—	27	—	—	19	240	—
		R	26	10	4	—	1	—	—	—	—	—	—	4	—
		U	711	286	1	2	1	—	—	27	—	—	19	236	—
5.	Baiswar :	T	7046	2478	420	245	—	—	8	21	26	20	6	42	280
		R	7040	2478	420	245	—	—	8	21	26	20	6	41	280
		U	6	—	—	—	—	—	—	—	—	—	—	1	—

(Contd.)

TABLE 3.3 : ***Contd.***

1	2		3	4	5	6	7	8	9	10	11	12	13	14	15
6.	Bhuiya :	T	6389	2752	1026	1361	4	93	27	53	113	2	2	67	163
		R	6284	2719	1026	1361	4	93	22	38	105	1	2	65	163
		U	105	33	—	—	—	—	5	15	8	1	—	2	—
7.	Chamar : (in lacs)	T	2.89	1.5379	0.568	1.572	183	212	6821	5674	769	341	1121	5086	3381
		R	2.75	1.11	0.32	0.62	163	201	6297	4909	648	220	814	2866	3312
		U	0.14	0.4279	0.248	0.952	20	11	524	765	121	121	307	2220	69
8.	Chero :	T	1586	6709	2796	3744	29	—	11	44	11	1	6	64	509
		R	1562	6698	2796	3744	29	—	11	40	11	1	6	58	509
		U	24	11	—	—	—	—	—	4	—	—	—	6	—
9.	Dhangar :	T	5109	1897	1000	518	1	—	45	19	—	1	—	11	110
		R	5105	1895	1000	518	1	—	45	19	—	1	—	10	110
		U	4	2	—	—	—	—	—	—	—	—	—	1	—
10.	**Dharkar :**	**T**	11634	5135	1306	2677	7	16	881	277	41	26	67	136	156
		R	10699	4810	1304	2651	6	16	824	183	26	5	38	66	143
		U	935	315	2	26	1	—	57	94	15	21	29	70	13
11.	**Dhobi :**	**T**	**7989**	6818	2575	2137	8	1	676	180	48	27	75	1090	538
		R	**6131**	6088	2560	2122	5	1	470	122	36	15	46	711	534
		U	**1858**	730	15	15	3	—	206	58	12	12	29	379	4
12.	**Dom :**	**T**	**1292**	**544**	34	81	12	—	118	103	—	2	27	167	5
		R	**660**	**293**	30	81	1	—	.98	26	—	—	9	47	5
		U	**632**	**251**	4	—	11	—	20	77	—	2	18	120	—

13. Dusadh :	T	9217	4203	1830	2327	6	—	146	110	15	7	54	147	108
	R	8928	4092	1377	2320	5	—	144	64	9	7	34	122	108
	U	289	111	3	7	1	—	2	46	6	—	20	25	—
14. Ghasiya :	T	1172	519	230	269	5	—	1	1	—	2	—	9	20
	R	1170	519	230	269	5	—	1	1	—	2	—	9	20
	U	2	—	—	—	—	—	—	—	—	—	—	—	—
15. Gond :	T	66198	27186	18494	7417	103	6	167	229	110	67	18	539	2082
	R	65446	26970	18478	7367	102	5	153	194	104	60	7	459	1803
	U	752	216	16	43	1	1	14	35	6	7	11	80	279
16. Hela :	T	644	244	13	14	—	—	19	18	1	1	15	161	2
	R	80	36	13	14	—	—	—	—	—	—	—	10	2
	U	564	208	—	—	—	—	19	18	1	1	15	151	—
17. Kharwar :	T	24893	3688	9581	4571	108	1	28	95	60	30	30	186	689
	R	24537	3593	9555	4550	108	1	21	79	55	30	25	170	689
	U	356	95	26	21	—	—	7	16	5	—	5	16	—
18. Khatik :	T	15430	5168	1065	920	93	2	1151	374	8	1018	54	179	215
	R	11280	3894	993	831	63	1	725	275	3	570	29	101	83
	U	4150	1274	72	89	30	1	426	99	5	448	25	78	132
19. Kol :	T	88311	24719	10544	32034	56	61	1004	1089	257	46	57	573	1173
	R	87858	24534	10541	31941	55	51	992	1070	252	41	49	542	1173
	U	453	185	3	93	1	10	12	19	5	5	8	31	—

(Contd.)

TABLE 3.3 : *Contd.*

1	2	3	4	5	6	7	8	9	10	11	12	13	14	15
20.	Kori :	T 3254	1358	457	530	2	1	84	158	7	33	22	64	4
		R 2615	1149	455	528	—	1	59	49	5	4	20	29	4
		U 639	209	2	2	2	—	25	109	2	29	2	35	—
21.	Korwa :	T 608	294	174	121	—	—	—	—	—	—	—	—	10
		R 608	294	174	121	—	—	—	—	—	—	—	—	10
		U —	—	—	—	—	—	—	—	—	—	—	—	—
22.	Majhwar :	T 4261	2037	1146	758	—	—	4	23	76	2	—	23	58
		R 4168	2009	1145	742	—	—	4	22	76	2	—	17	58
		U 93	28	1	16	—	—	—	1	—	—	—	6	—
23.	Mushar :	T 12031	6124	620	3981	3	34	737	314	73	123	9	230	135
		R 11587	5942	616	3956	—	34	635	288	62	123	7	221	135
		U 444	182	4	25	3	—	102	26	11	—	2	9	—
24.	Nat :	T 1224	496	120	261	—	—	45	13	3	23	1	27	12
		R 1150	475	119	254	—	—	45	11	2	16	1	24	11
		U 74	21	1	7	—	—	—	2	1	7	—	3	1
25.	Pankha :	T 2378	1044	452	482	—	3	19	2	8	9	—	65	18
		R 2159	962	450	463	—	2	8	1	2	3	—	37	16
		U 219	82	2	19	—	1	11	1	6	6	—	28	2

26. Parahiya :	T	526	211	116	88	1	—	2	8	2	8	9	—	9
	R	485	197	113	78	—	—	2	8	1	2	3	—	9
	U	41	14	3	10	1	—	—	—	1	6	6	—	—
27. Pasi :	T	23238	8716	2092	2857	33	22	1679	1142	66	52	242	479	131
	R	21672	8144	2083	2803	31	18	1592	1033	37	24	201	320	131
	U	1566	572	9	54	2	4	87	109	29	28	41	159	—
28. Patari :	T	651	269	164	88	3	—	1	2	1	—	1	6	10
	R	639	267	164	88	3	—	1	1	1	—	1	5	10
	U	12	2	—	—	—	—	—	1	—	—	—	1	—

Note : T = Total; R = Rural; U = Urban

the main Scheduled Castes found in Sonbhadra district and in the rest of the State as well. These castes were, by and large, suffering from the stigma of untouchability in the past. A profile of these castes has been given in tables 3.3 and 3.4. The present status of all these groups including those of tribal origins is that of Scheduled Castes under the Presidential Order issued in 1950.

Tracing their history back to the earlier part of this century, the Mirzapur District Gazetteer (1911) described nineteen groups as "aboriginal tribes". These were the Kol, Majhwar, Kharwar, Biyar, Gond, Bind, Dharkar, Chero, Pankha, Baiswar, Bhuiya, Dhangar, Bhuinyar, Pahri, Agaria, Korwa, Pathari, Parahiya and Ghasia. The Gazetteer of 1988 uses such terms as 'aboriginal tribes', "Dravidian Tribes' and 'Non-Aryan Tribes' for all of them excepting Pahri.

The entire area now forming the Sonbhadra district was a Scheduled District under the provisions of the Scheduled Districts Act, 1874 which dealt with areas of tribal concentration throughout the British India. This law vested wide powers of legislation by simple executive orders in the Executive (India 1962). The Government of India Excluded and Partially Excluded Areas Order, 1936 issued under Section 91 of the Government of India Act, 1935 listed "the portion of the Mirzapur District south of Kaimur range" (BAJSS 1951) as a Partially Excluded Area. Thus, the area had a special status before Independence. But, the tribal people living therein were not listed as 'backward tribes' as per the 13th Schedule to the Government of India (Provincial Legislative Assemblies Order), 1935 (BAJSS 1951 : 32-38) as they had adopted widely the traits of the Hindu castes living around them.

Our Constitution includes provisions for the Scheduled Castes, the Scheduled Tribes and the Scheduled Areas (relatable to the former Partially Excluded Areas). The Scheduled Castes and the Scheduled Tribes were to be declared through Presidential Orders, in consultation with the State Government concerned while Scheduled Areas could be so declared through Presidential orders at the initiative of the Government of India (Saksena 1981). However, the Government of U.P. used this opportunity to bring about 'normalisation of administration' in its Partially Excluded Areas. They did not agree to the scheduling of any tribes and consequently no Scheduled Areas, contrary to some specific provisions proposing Scheduled Tribes and also Scheduled areas for the State in the Draft Constitution of February 1948. (India 1948 : 172-73, 205; Rao 1968 : 578). Later in 1955 the State Government veered round to the view that U.P. should have Scheduled Tribes and sent proposals to change the status of thirteen 'tribal' groups (almost all residing in Sonbhadra and the adjoining districts) from Scheduled Castes to Scheduled Tribes. This proposal has, however, remained pending with the Government of India since then, not because of any lack of merit in the case (Lok Sabha 1969) but because the proposed amendments to the lists of the Scheduled Castes and the Scheduled Tribes from all over India are too controversial for easy adoption in the Parliament. Five tribal communities in the hills and the terai areas were declared Scheduled Tribes through a Presidential Order in June 1967 as there was no change of status involved in their case, which needs Parliament's approval under Articles 341 and 342.

The tribal groups in question meanwhile continue with the status of Scheduled Castes. Subsequently the Government of U.P. have, however, started treating them as "non-Scheduled Tribes" allowing "all facilities due to Scheduled Tribes" (Hasan 1985). But this approach obviously cannot go beyond provision of some extra funds for the schemes among these groups. The benefits of special funds under Article 275(1) of the Constitution for the Scheduled Tribes and reservation in government services cannot be made available for them. The schemes launched for them were mainly educational, viz. stipends,

TABLE 3.4 : **Literacy and Education among Scheduled Castes in Mirzapur District—1981**

Sl. No.	Caste	Population	Literates		Literates without educational level	Primary and middle	Matriculation /Inter including Diploma	Graduate and above
			Number	Percentage				
1.	Agaria	6530	89	1.4	59	28	1	1
2.	Baheliya	678	104	15.5	39	53	12	—
3.	Baiga	8296	113	1.3	85	26	2	—
4.	Baiswar	7046	1282	13.2	595	556	109	22
5.	Balmiki	737	208	28.2	93	91	22	—
6.	Bhuiya	6389	184	2.8	96	74	14	—
7.	Chamar	288580	27078	9.3	12820	10250	3445	553
8.	Chero	15086	477	3.2	322	135	17	3
9.	Dhangar	5109	329	6.4	189	127	13	—
10.	Dharkar	11634	700	6.0	279	285	36	—
11.	Dhobi	7989	2468	30.9	1157	1023	251	37
12.	Dom	1292	110	8.5	49	52	9	—
13.	Dusadh	9217	1047	11.4	538	396	105	8
14.	Ghasia	1172	34	2.8	15	19	—	—
15.	Gond	66198	4514	6.8	2486	1744	260	24

16.	Hela	644	191	29.6	78	82	24	7
17.	Kharwar	34893	1834	5.3	1215	536	78	5
18.	Khatik	15430	1654	10.7	804	656	166	28
19.	Kol	88311	2437	2.8	1886	446	91	14
20.	Kori	3254	625	18.3	258	304	58	5
21.	Korwa	608	7	1.1	7	—	—	—
22.	Majhwar	4261	476	11.2	352	112	12	—
23.	Musahar	12031	184	1.5	131	48	5	—
24.	Nat	1224	85	6.9	42	30	13	—
25.	Pankha	2378	200	8.4	101	85	13	1
26.	Parhaiya	526	20	3.8	15	5	—	—
27.	Pasi	23238	3204	13.8	1405	1373	358	68
28.	Patari	651	66	10.1	28	34	4	—

residential *ashram* schools, and an industrial training institute. Hasan (1985) is of the view that "normal administration is causing havoc in their life style, culture, customary laws and above all to their economy, and the application of all the general laws to the area, which would not have happened if these were Scheduled Areas". Considering what has been happening to the land rights and the neglect of the area and the developmental needs of the tribals this observation is not unfounded.

Majumdar was the first anthropologist to study the tribal people of U.P., particularly those residing in the Mirzapur district. His studies in this area spanned a period of almost two decades. Speaking of U.P. tribes, he says "the main concentration of tribal population is in the Mirzapur district which is adjacent to Chhota Nagpur Plataeu, and bounded in the south and south-west by a number of feudatory states which harbours quite significant number of tribal groups. The policy of *Laissez Faire* followed by state authorities with respect to tribal populations, has maintained the solidarity, also the isolation of the tribes and the conditions found there offer a striking contrast to those existing in other parts . . ." (Majumdar 1944). However, the conditions in the area today present a picture at variance from what he had observed and the basic factors responsible for such a situation are the introduction of normal administration followed by rapid industrialisation.

The ethnographic notes on the tribal communities in Sonbhadra which were prepared in the course of this study and also the case studies, that follow, throw light on how far the tribal people in the area possess the characteristics of tribes and the extent to which they have been acculturated to occupy sociologically a position akin to castes. Twelve major communities hav been described in the section that follows.

The Agaria

The Agaria, a small tribal community found only in this area of the State "approximate very closely to allied Dravidian tribes such as the Korwa and the Parahias" (Misra 1988). Majumdar (1960) regards them and Korwa as the most primitive elements in the population here, the former speaking a dialect akin to the Mundari. However, in the neighbouring Madhya Pradesh where they are treated as Scheduled Tribes, the origins of the Agaria are related to the Gond (Tiwari 1984). The Uttar Pradesh Agaria believe that more than a century ago they had migrated to this area from Rewa, settling down first in the village of Khairahi in Dudhi pargana.

The Agaria are traditionally iron-smelters and continue to function as the *Lohar* (blacksmiths) for both tribals and non-tribals of the area among whom they are welcomed (Majumdar 1960). Through their primitive methods of mining and smelting, the Agaria have been utilising the iron ore even with a poor percentage of iron content. They make utensils and crude iron implements used in agriculture and forest operations. They also work as labourers to supplement their income and some have agricultural lands, like the ones found in our sample. However, those who practised the traditional occupation either moved from one village to another selling the iron implements, or one or two families are seen settled down in larger and important villages. Thus, they are a semi-nomadic tribal group with a strong symbiotic link with other tribes and castes in the area. The Agaria are among the poorest section of the tribal population. They have played a more important role in the economy of the Dudhi area as compared to the Singrauli area where some migrants of the Lohar caste had settled down because the Raja of Singrauli provided facilities to them. However, these families had mostly taken to carpentry and did not practice blacksmithy.

The Agaria regard themselves as Hindus but till

recent times they were not worshipping the common Hindu deities. They depend upon the services of Baiga tribals as priests and medicine men. In the month of *Aghan* and *Pusa* they worshipped their tribe's main deity, Lohasurdevi, the goddess of iron. The offerings were made through the Baiga priest.

They do not have exogamous subdivisions based on totem but the septs (*gotra*) are very much there to regulate marriage relations. Their life cycle ceremonies are simple. At birth an elderly woman conducts the delivery and *chhati* (sixth day) and *barhi* (twelfth day) ceremonies are observed. Marriages are performed during the rainy season, unlike other communities, obviously because the traditional work of iron smelting is not carried out then. The Baiga has a role in the marriage ceremonies and the rituals begin with digging some earth from the hearth made for iron smelting and offering it to the bride's mother. Bride price in kind is practised. Marriage rites are performed by their *behnoi* (sister's husband). The dead are cremated.

Educationally the Agaria are very backward with a literacy rate of only 1.3 per cent, in 1981.

The Bhuiya

The Bhuiya are a Dravidian tribe and they claim descent from the sons of two *rishis*, known as Bhad and Mahesh and for this reason call themselves Rishasian Bhuiya. This legend asserts their kinship with the Mushar and Bhuinyar. Their chief deity is the Hindu Kali, who had doubtlessly succeeded some aboriginal goddess, but they also worship through the Baiga, the village gods and *Dharti Mata*. They have a special tribal hero named Nadu Bir. Most Bhuiyas are hereditary ploughmen, but some are engaged in catechu making and hence known as Khairahas. They are quiet, industrious and simple (Drake-Brockman 1911).

They are found in Dudhi and Singrauli parganas of

Dudhi tahsil. Amongst the tribals, they occupy the lowest position analogous to the Chamar in Hindu caste hierarchy (Majumdar 1960). Their dwellings are small and generally at one end of the village. They are experts in making traps and shooting with bows and arrows. They used to roam about in the jungles for game and collection of forest produce like gum and honey and cutting of bamboo and timber and fuel wood. Now, most of them are engaged as agriculture labour and some are cultivators.

At child birth, usually an elderly female conducts the delivery and *chhati* (sixth day) and *barhi* (twelfth day) ceremonies are observed. Widow remarriage and divorce are permissible. Marriages are of two types, *biyah* and *sagai* as found in other castes of the region. *biyah* is between the spouses not married earlier, while *Sagai* is the term for a marriage where one or both parties are widow/widower/divorcee. Bride price was the norm but it is not strictly practised now. The dead are cremated.

They have faith in ghosts and spirits. A Baiga is consulted while taking up any activity in the forest or in agriculture. They also observe Hindu festivals like Holi, Diwali, Nag-panchami, etc., besides regular worship at village *devsthan*, *Baigadih* and of other objects.

Now they are primarily engaged in agriculture in many ways: as cultivator, share cropper, *halwaha* or labour. Besides collecting forest produce like *mahua, ber, amla*, gum, honey, and fuel wood, they also keep cattle needed in agriculture. Both men and women work as labourers for big cultivators. They are known for their honesty and hard labour. They are also employed for cutting of bamboo and timber trees in the forests by the local contractors. Most of them are stated to move from one place to another in search of work, but due to extensive clearance of forests and restrictions on access to forests they have been leading a more settled life.

The Bhuiya are now relatively more conscious about

education and send their children to schools. In 1961, the literacy figure for the tribe was 3.14 but a limited survey in 1982 indicated that 33 per cent Bhuiya families were sending their male children to schools. Girls' education was not encouraged because they were usually detained at home for doing family chores. Just 43 per cent of Bhuiya households possessed land against the average of 67 per cent for all tribals. A large number of Bhuiya households (72%) did not possess any cattle wealth. Among them, 18 per cent earned their livelihood from cultivation, 1.20 per cent from agriculture labour, 78.21 per cent from non-agricultural labour, 2.03 per cent from service and 0.56 per cent from animal husbandry. Female participation in economic activities was highest among the Bhuiya, i.e. 44 per cent as against the average of 40 per cent for all tribals. Two room dwelling units were found among 50 per cent households of Bhuiya.

In the Singrauli area their economic position was better. Here many Bhuiya families used to maintain 30-40 cattle for dairying and agricultural operations and they were also owners of small agricultural holdings.

The Chero (Baiga)

The Chero are popularly known as the Baiga. They are included in the list of Scheduled Castes in U.P. whereas in M.P. amd Bihar they are Scheduled Tribes. They are undoubtedly of Dravidian stock, and are probably a branch of the well-known Kol tribe with whom they enjoy connubiality. As they exist today they are a community of labourers and cultivators. Their great god is Gansam Deo besides Raja Chandol and Bariyar Sah and they are ancestor worshippers also (Drake-Brockman 1911).

They are the oldest inhabitants and claim that once they were rulers of the Dudhi area. They engage in *purohitai* (priesthood) and *ojhai* (sorcery) among the tribal people of the area. They are considered experts in controlling all types of ghosts and spirits who are propitiated by the tribals, being endowed with supernatural powers. They are also known as Parhaiyas. They also perform rituals like *tersuiya* before sowing which ensures that the crop is good. They also practise exorcising of the 'demons' of diseases among the tribal people and are in demand in times of troubles and epidemics. It is a source of income for them. They also perform rituals to seek protection from evil spirits responsible for epidemics and natural calamities overtaking the village (Hasan 1982).

They are quite industrious and proficient in making traps, pitfalls and hunting with bow and arrow. Their speed of climbing trees on any alarm of animals is proverbial. Many of them have taken up work as masons also and in 1960 some of the families were stated to have worked in the construction of the Rihand dam. By and large, they work as labourers or ploughmen (*halwaha*). Like other tribes, they are also engaged in cultivation as cultivator or agriculture labour. Collection of forest produce like *chironji, ber, amla, mahua*, honey, gum, fuel wood, etc. was another source of income because they were known as masters of forests, having superior powers of controlling evil spirits residing there. But now this facility is hardly available due to restrictions in the forests.

In Singrauli area they were agriculturists and keepers of cattle. Besides *purohitai*, they used to maintain a good number of milch cattle as well as bullocks. Dairying was practised and it is said that even poor families used to maintain a mininum of 30-40 cattle. Now this trade has declined and they are found mostly as labourers or cultivator.

Besides regular worship of tribal gods and malevolent and benevolent spirits and ghosts they have started worshipping Hindu gods and goddesses. A Chero in Rajkhar village three kms. from Dudhi worships both Shivaling and goddess Kali. They observe Hindu fairs and festivals like Holi, Diwali, Dasahra, etc. with enthusiasm. They occupy a distinct place in the religious world of tribals.

Literacy among them was extremely low (1.3) in 1981. However, there has been some change since their children are now attending schools. Some boys have passed High School, Intermediate and B.A. A few have taken up teaching in the local schools.

As regards life cycle ceremonies, no ceremony is performed during pregnancy and at childbirth. Usually elderly females of the community attend to delivery. *chatti* (sixth day) and *barhi* (twelfth day) ceremonies are observed. Marriage within the caste is a must but *kuri* exogamy is the rule. Marriage of boy with a virgin is known as *biyah* and if either of the spouse is widow/ widower or divorcee it is termed as *sagai*. Three stages of marriages are usually observed in the region. The first is *shadi* (actual marriage) when bride comes to groom's house and stays for 3-4 days and then she is sent back to her parents' house; thereafter *gauna* (second marriage) takes place when bride comes to her husband's house for another 3-4 days and again sent back to her parents. Finally after *donga*, the wife comes to stay with her husband's family. These three stages are prevalent because early marriage were practised for both boys and girls. Marriagesare usually performed in the month of *Phagun* and *Baisakh*. The custom of bride price or dowry is not prevalent among them. Gifts in kind are however given. Child marriage is practised and polygyny is also permissible. In marriages a *mandap* is erected in which nine poles are used, instead of five as amongst other tribals. The ceremony of *matkarwa*—performing a *havan* in the centre of the *mandap* after bringing earth from the nearby agricultural fields to that place for erecting the pole is also performed by the Baiga. Now, *barat* (groom's party) is taken to the bride's place for which local musical bands are engaged but in the past *dola* (bride's party) used to come to the groom's house for marriage.

They cremate their dead.

The Baiga have been adversely affected by displacements. On account of it they have lost their agricultural land and agriculture labour and their traditional *purohitai* work on the occasion of different agricultural activities and other ceremonies too has ended. Now they have become landless and compelled to engage in odd work. In Ambedkar Nagar and another settlement at Rakhbandhi groups of Baiga families were found to be living in temporary sheds and in dire poverty.

The Gond

The Gond are a numerically large tribe in the district. They are also called Majhwar or Manjhi. In M.P. and Bihar they are a Scheduled Tribe. The latter name is derived from the Sanskrit word *Madhya* or middle, and is said to mean either the holders of the middle land or more probably leader or headman. The Gond are divided into atleast a dozen sub-tribes, inhabiting several states in Central India.

In Sonbhadra, they are divided into five exogamous subdivisions known as Poiya, Tekam, Marai, Oika and Olku, each of which includes a number of totemistic septs said to have been derived from a Gond who had five sons (Drake-Brockman 1911). The Gond or Majhi remember their original place being in some part of Sarangarh, Raigarh district of M.P. Many legends establishing their relationship with Gond rulers in pre-independent India are still passed down from generation to generation. They have their own priests from amongst the Pathari, an offshoot of Gond. Socially and economically they are better off than the other tribes, their status as 'rulers of the jungle' and many former states being acknowledged.

The Gond are engaged in agriculture either as cultivators of small and medium sized holdings or as agricultural labourers. In 1961, about 82.85 per cent of their working population depended on agriculture, 10.36

per cent were agricultural labourers, 2.78 per cent pursued household industries and 2.41 per cent were in 'other services'. Under household industry basket, mats, *soops*, etc. are also made by them.

In the past, they had a dominant position in land management of the area, particularly Dudhi. Here the land management was with *supurdars* many of whom were Gond. People used to take land for cultivation from them. *Supurdari* system continued till the abolition of zamindari. In early fifties, immigrants from Bihar and adjoining areas came for business and settled down permanently taking land of the tribals. Some of them also served in lower positions in the revenue and police departments and took advantage of their position in obtaining lands. The migrants also turned into money-lenders and exploited the simple and ignorant tribals taking full advantage of poor crops, drought and famine. For instance, Mangal Majhi, great grandson of Nankoo Majhi, who was *supurdar* of the area around Dudhi had to part with 18 *bighas* of land in this manner to a Bania (Majumdar 1960).

In agricultural practices, Gonds like others, employ a Baiga priest on different occasions. In the event of crop diseases also he is consulted and performs rituals to ward them off. The Baiga used to get five seers of grain from each agricultural family and used to serve 4-5 villages (Majumdar 1960). All agricultural work like ploughing, manuring, sowing/transplanting and harvesting were initiated only after the rituals were performed by the Baiga, as a part of which he sacrificed hen/goat and offered liquor to the deity Mahadani. The practices continue among the agriculturists. The forest was an additional source to supplement their income. Minor forest produce like *ber, mahua, chironji,* gum, honey, fuel wood and building material were available to them. But now with the rigid restrictions in the forests and reduction in forest area they hardly get anything.

Hunting is now totally forbidden. Cattle were kept in large numbers but its pedigree was not good. These were mainly kept as status symbol, as well as to obtain cow-dung for manure and fuel. In Singrauli area the cattle were of a better quality and the land was fertile. But now they face difficulties in rearing cattle.

The Gond like other tribals build their houses in the field and thus their houses are at some distance from one another. The houses are usually *kaccha,* made of mud walls, with thatched or tiled roofing. An average house contains several rooms, space for kitchen, a large courtyard and some space for keeping cattle.

No ceremony is performed before the delivery of the child. The expectant mother is kept in a separate small room known as *sauri* and male members are not allowed to enter in it. A local *dai,* usually a Chamar woman, is called for conducting delivery and massaging the mother and the new born for six days. Birth pollution is observed for six days and with the *chhati* ceremony on sixth day the pollution ends. Child marriages are not practised. Two types of marriages are in vogue among them also, *biyah* and *sagai.* Marriage by exchange is also practised. Marriage has three stages i.e., *shadi, gauna* and *donga* or *rauna.* These are usually performed in the months of *Magh, Phalgun* and *Baisakh* and sometimes in *Jeth* also. Bride price in kind was the common practice but now dowry is fast coming in vogue. *Gauna* is performed usually after one or one and a half years of marriage. The rules of intra-community marriage and *gotra* exogamy are strictly followed. The Gonds used to take the services of Pathari priests previously but now they have been replaced by the Brahmin priests. But the Baiga still performs the ceremony of *matkorwa* in the *mandap.* Among them a *bhala* (spear) is fixed in the *mandap* and the groom and bride keep swords on their shoulders and take circumbulation of the *bhala,* five times. When the bride comes to the groom's house she is made to sit and women make a parting of her hair over which mustard oil mixed with *haldi* (turmeric) powder is poured and if this liquid flows from the parting to the middle of nose, she is considered faithful to her husband. Marriage party (*barat*) was earlier accompanied by local bands played by the Chamar or Dharkar. But now with the influence of urban culture they prefer to go for professional bands, illumination, etc. making marriage a costly affair.

The Gonds believe strongly in ghosts and spirits and these are appeased on appropriate occasions with the help of the *ojha*, the Pathari priests and the Baiga. Burha Deo is their supreme god whose worship is compulsory on initiating any work or function. They observe festivals of Holi, Diwali and Nagpanchami. In Holi the custom of cutting *sambat* (cutting a branch of *semal* (*Bambrax ceiba*) tree) is done by the Baiga and then Holi is celebrated with gaiety. The better status of the Gond is indicated by the practice that they can throw colour on the Brahman and Thakur also. They have great faith in magic which is of two types, benevolent and malevolent. They are most afraid of *dains* and *churail* and consider it imperative to appease them for peaceful living.

The traditional *birdari panchayat* headed by the *Chaudhary* used to play a vital role in resolving tribal disputes related to marriages, sex-relations, etc. The jurisdiction of a *birdari panchayat* depended on the population and nearness of their villages. Sometimes village level *panchayats* included two-three villages. The bigger *panchayat* for the area was known as *jawar panchayat*. The influence of the *panchayat* and its organisation have suffered adversely in the last few years.

Literacy among the Gond was low (5.1 per cent in 1961) and among the females it was negligible. But now they have started sending their children to schools specially the government residential schools (*ashram* schools). There is one such school for girls as well. Now, there are a few graduates and technical diploma-holders among them. Awareness for their interests has increased and a few Gond leaders have joined and led agitations for land rights like the *Bhoomi Haqdari Morcha* and literacy compaign. The outgoing M.L.A. also belongs to this community.

The Gond also take pride in mentioning that in the early fifties a popular reformation movement, was launched by a Gond woman, Raj Mohini Devi. This movement was a great success. She was considered a *Devi* (goddess). Her teachings were simple : (1) Live an unostentatious and honest life, and speak truth; (2) Do not harm the weak, even animals; (3) Give up liquor and meat; (4) Practice personal hygiene, viz. a daily bath, clean clothes and daily cleaning of houses; and (5) Devotion to God and spending some time in religious activities like *bhajan* and *kirtan*, etc. Her teaching had a profound influence on the tribals and they gave up non-vegetarian food, liquor and followed her lessons of personal hygiene and cleanliness of houses. In several villages, a *chabutra* was raised in her name where people assembled and sang *bhajans*. But her influence did not last long. About 1957, the movement suffered a setback and the followers started reverting to their old ways (Majumdar 1960).

The Kharwar

Numerically the Kharwar constitute a sizeable group of tribals in the district. In the adjoining State of M.P. and Bihar they are listed as Scheduled Tribes. Their name is derived either from their occupation as makers of catechu from the *khair* tree or from their traditional home Khairagarh. According to Santal legends, the two tribes, Kharwar and Santal are identical and if this is accepted Khairagarh must be the place of that name in the district of Hazaribagh. The Mirzapur tradition, however, seems to point to a place of the same name to the south or west, in which case Khairagarh must be identified with the state of that name in Chhattisgarh or with the Khairagarh tahsil of Allahabad district. Some of them call themselves Surajbansis, others say they are a mixed race that originated in the time of King Ben and call themselves Benbansi Rajputs. Of "all the aboriginal tribes of the district, they are the most deeply tinged with Hinduism. They have four exogamous subdivisions known as Surajbansi, Dualbandhi, Patabandhi and Benbansi and one endogamous subdivision called the Khairaha" (Drake-Brockman 1911).

In the mid-century, the Kharwar were found to be at different levels of cultural development. One branch, the Surajbansi Kharwar was engaged in large scale production of catechu by idigenous methods while Dualbandhi and Patabandhi Kharwars considered this occupation as low and degrading. The Surajabanshi Kharwar called themselves as Khairahi and claimed to be a separate caste. They used to assemble in the forests of Dudhi tahsil in the month of February and take *khair* forests on lease (*patta*) where they erected temporary workshops for manufacturing catechu and huts for their living. Other groups of Khairwars were agriculturists and also collected fruits and herbs from forests. Both men and women worked, in cultivation. However, ploughing was done by males only and other works like sowing, weeding, cutting, etc. were shared by both sexes. Collection of minor forest produce, viz., *mahua, ber, chironji, fuel-wood* was undertaken to supplement their income. As high as 83.5 per cent of their working population depended on agriculture, 12.9 per cent worked in the fields as labourers and 3.6 per cent in household industry, livestock, etc. (Census 1961).

Cattle were kept in large numbers as grazing facilities were available in the forests. These were mainly kept not for dairy but for agriculture and cow-dung which was used as manure. Milch cattle were of small pedigree in this area but in Singrauli cattle rearing was done on a large scale and their cows were famous. Even poor families used to maintain 30 to 40 cattle. Agriculture was traditional and the use of chemical fertilizers, improved seeds, etc. was unknown to them. Irrigation too was scanty and depended mostly on monsoon. Two crops, *rabi* and *kharif* were grown.

They also undertook work as labourer in forests. A forest official said that in this area the relations of tribals with the forest department have been good, barring the recent agitation for rights over their land. Forest Department provided them employment throughout the year. In April-May a large number took up work of collection of *tendu* leaves, in June for upturning the earth of pits made for afforestation, in July-August for plantation activities and in the rest of the year for levelling, repair and construction of forest roads, clearing of forests, etc.

Kharwars have lived in mixed villages with other castes and tribes. Village boundaries were big because houses were built at some distance from one another, in the field—a normal pattern in this area. The houses were *kutcha* with mud walls and tiled or thatched roofing, consisting of 2-3 rectangular rooms with little ventilation, verandah, kitchen and a courtyard, along with sufficient open space for keeping cattle.

The Kharwar call themselves Hindus, but previously they did not worship any of the common Hindu gods, except the Sun, whom they appeased in time of trouble and to whom the householder bowed when he left his house in the morning. The tribal deities were Jualamukhi Devi and Raja Lakhan. Other local deities were Mahadev, Raja Chandol and Dharti-mata or mother earth, usually worshipped in association with the collective village gods in the month of *Baisakh*. Later the Kharwars of better class had, besides other Hindu customs, adopted the practice of making offerings in the name of the dead (*shraddha*). Many of them have now started wearing a sacred thread and claiming Rajput origins.

The Kharwar are superstitious and have great faith

in ghosts and spirits. A protracted illness is attributed to the wrath of evil spirits and they resort to the services of *ojha* (medicine man) for driving them out. Good and bad omens are followed and some magical practices are also prevalent.

In agricultural activities the role of Baiga was very important. The Baiga performs *havan* (oblations) in the name of Mahadani at the time of ploughing new land, burning of manure in the fields, sowing, etc. and also sacrifices a cock and offers drops of liquor. The Baiga is paid in kind and some cash for his services. Similarly before undertaking work in the forest, the Baiga performed a ritual for the appeasement of forest spirits.

No ceremony is performed during pregnancy. At child birth the services of a Chamar midwife (*dai*) is taken for six days till pollution lasts. On the sixth day (*chhati*) the mother and child are given a bath. Like other tribes Kharwar marriages are also performed in three stages, *shadi, gauna* and *donga* or *rauna* and payment of bride-price in kind was common. Tilak ceremony was not prevalent among them. But now the custom of *Tilak* is becoming common. Child marriages are not preferred. The Baiga has an important role in marriage also. He is called for making the marriage-booth (*mandap*) and performing the ceremony of *matkorwa*. The marriage rites are performed by a Brahmin priest. Divorce is permissible and marriage with divorced women is known as *Sagai* which is solemnised in a simple way.

In early fifties the Kharwar too were influenced by the Raj Mohini Devi movement described earlier. The influence of this social and reformation movement started waning after the late fifties among the Kharwar as well. However they state that they continue to attach importance to personal hygiene and cleanliness of their dwellings.

Literacy among the Kharwar was as low as 3.6 per cent in 1961. Now they are sending their boys to schools but female education is not encouraged. Some of them have since passed High School, Intermediate and B.A. examinations and a few have acquired technical diplomas also.

They had a strong *Birdari Panchayat* headed by *Mahto* at the turn of the century and in the mid-century. At village level or for groups of two-three villages smaller *panchayats* were there. For important decisions a *Jawar panchayat* covering eight to ten villages was also called. The panchayat dealt with cases of theft, illicit sex offences, violation of caste norms, divorce, family quarrels, etc. This organisation has considerably weakened now.

The Kol

The Kol are the largest tribal group in U.P. In M.P. they are a Scheduled Tribe. They are mostly found in the Robertsganj tahsil, and in the adjoining districts of Mirzapur, Allahabad and Banda.

They are emigrants from a place called Kutali in the territories of the Bardi Raja in Rewa state. They name one Nanhu as their ancestor and, like the Musahars, have a tribal temple at Pipri near Chunar, which is the shrine of Birmha Devi. Their name is probably derived from *Ho* which means "a man" in the pure Kol dialect. The customs of the Kol have now become deeply tinged with Hinduism. They have shaken off the elaborate system of totemic septs still found among the Munda of Bengal and have adopted a structure of *subdivisions,* endogamous *kuris* or *gotras*. They are divided into seven such *gotras* (Drake-Brockman 1911). Most of the Kol of Mirzapur are Rajbansis while those of Allahabad and Banda are Thakurias and Ravatias.

They now worship Hindu gods and goddesses such as Rama, Hanuman and Shankar Bhagwan besides their own deities namely Banaspatimata, Phoolmati Devi, Dulhadeo, Babadeva, Bhagat, Bhairon, Mata Sharda, Subban and Amina. The Kol also worship demons and spirits and the souls of the dead. Their chief god is Raja Lakhan. He sometimes has a crude shrine of his own but is generally believed to inhabit the village *bargad* tree and is worshipped by the head of the family.

They have a strong traditional *panchayat,* headed by the *Chaudhari*. The *Chaudhari* is assisted by a *Deevan* and has at his disposal a number of *sipahi* who work as process servers. The *panchayat* is called for settlement of disputes and its decisions are rarely challenged. Now this institution has been over-shadowed by the statutory panchayats and shifts in residence due to their movement for labour work.

The Kol is one of the poorest tribes. They have little land with the result that they have to work as agricultural or industrial labourers to earn their livelihood. Most of them are indebted to the money-lenders due to which they are often held in debt-bondage, particularly in the Banda district (Hasan 1982). They also work for the contractors in the stone-quarries of Allahabad, Mirzapur and Sonbhadra often under a system of debt bondage.

They generally live in huts which are small and huddled together.

Educationally they are still very backward and had a literacy level of less than 3 per cent in 1981 with negligible female literacy. Several residential schools were set up during the eighties to encourage education among their children.

The Chamar

The Chamar is the largest Scheduled Caste of U.P. and Sonbhadra district as well. Their traditional occupation has been connected with skinning of dead animals and other leather work including making of shoes. But now this work is done by some of the families only and, by and large, they are labourers and marginal cultivators in the rural areas. They are treated as untouchables and occupy almost the lowest position in the caste hierarchy.

Labourers for different agricultural operations employed for ploughing, sowing, harvesting, irrigation, land reclamation, cutting of fuel wood, etc. are mostly from this caste. Women also work as labourers, besides being the traditional midwife (*dai*) for all castes.

In Singrauli state they are stated to have been given patronage like other serving artisan castes. In Chilkadand, some displaced families of this caste said that before displacement they were owners of holdings ranging from 10 to 25 acres of land and on this basis their caste people got regular employment in the NTPC, as well as house-plots. A similar position was also reported from NCL and Bijpur area which shows that in due course they had acquired land for cultivation through their hard labour. They used to keep a good number of cattle before displacement.

Many Chamars who worked as agricultural labourers called *halwahas* or as sharecropper were the worst sufferers of displacement. They did not get any job and are depending on daily labour which is not always available. Many women and children of this caste besides others are seen picking coals at railway track, roads, etc. In the past this section was occupied in grazing of cattle and collection of forest produce from the jungle. They also work in brick kilns.

Marriage ceremony was performed by the *behnoi* (sister's husband) but now a Brahmin priest is called. Widow remarriage and divorce are permissible. Bride price in kind is practised.

They have a *birdari panchayat* headed by a *Chaudhary*. It deals with cases of theft, social offence, violation of caste-rules, family quarrels, sex offences, etc. Now its role has declined. They observe Hindu festivals and have faith in magic and sorcery as well. Baiga/Ojha is consulted in the event of illness, crop diseases, and for driving away evil spirits.

The Dharkar

Dharkars are a sub-caste of the eastern Doms, and are also known as Bentbansis, because they traditionally do cane (*bent*) work. The Dharkars are included in the list of Scheduled Castes. Bamboo is 'a sort of totem' and is treated with great respect by the Dharkar. They call themselves Hindus but have a special pantheon of their own, as well. Pahar Pando is a mountain god and Durasin, Banhiya Bir and Deonath are deified heroes. Agarmati Bhawani, the goddess of blazing charcoal is a female divinity. They also worship Dulha Deo and Parcho Pir. They have a very strong 'tribal council'. Drake-Brockman's (1911) account depicts them as a tribal group.

The Dharkar have four sections (*kuri*), viz. Aril, Neoriya, Dauriha and Nagarha named after different varieties of bamboo. Aril is said to be the name of a fine kind of bamboo used in making winnowing fans, baskets, sieves, etc.; Neuriya is said to be derived from *newar* the young soft bamboo; Dauriha is said to have derived its name from *Dauiwa*, a strong hard bamboo and Naharha from *nagar* a very high thick bamboo. These sections intermarry on equal terms except the Aril, which is the highest and with which others practise hypergamy (Misra 1988). A majority of Dharkars are now engaged in labour work, agricultural or non-agricultural, and soms families own lands. They also collect minor forest produce as they frequently visit the jungles for cutting of bamboo for their occupation of basketry.

Literacy has been low among the Dharkars (6.0% in 1981) but a trend of sending their children to schools has now started.

At child birth, elderly female of the family usually attends to the delivery. Marriages are performed by sister's husband or *maan* (*behnoi*) but now some lowly Brahmin priests are also being called. *maan*, the term used for sister's husband is derived from the Hindu word *manya*, meaning 'respected'.

The Baiga is consulted by them also for performing rituals related to agriculture and forest activities.

They celebrate Hindu festivals like Holi, Dewali, Nag-Panchmi. But they also worship Dulha Deo and Panhan Pir.

The Dharkar caste *panchayat* is powerful and its decisions are adhered to.

The Panika

Numerically, the Panika is a small Scheduled Caste in the district. In M.P. they are treated as a Scheduled Tribe. 'The male members work as weavers and are employed as watchmen. Living in the south of the district they are known differently as Panka, Panika, or Pankiya and Kotwar, the last of which means keeper or porter of a castle'. The name Panka or Panika is usually taken to be derived from *panik* which means the elastic bow which the weaver use to extend the cloth as it is woven. Though they have lost their totemistic septs in Mirzapur, still their appearance clearly indicates their connection with the Majhwars (Drake-Brockman 1911).

Like Gonds they are divided into a number of exogamous *kuris* such as Gaigual, Bajar, Dakehhal, Teria, Parvar, etc. Their Baiga (tribal priests) come from the Chero tribe. The Brahmin too is called for their religious ceremonies. Most of them are either small cultivators or landless labourers. They are also employed as watchmen. Fishing, hunting and the collection of minor forest produce are their other means of subsistence (Misra 1988).

In the past their traditional occupation was weaving and coarse cloth produced by them was used by the other tribes and the local people. But with the availability of mill cloth in the region, their traditional occupation was gradually abandoned. In some villages like Rajkhar and Bidar near Dudhi town and in Singrauli pargana weaving of cloth continued as a subsidiary means of livelihood and cloth prepared by the Panika was a must in the marriage of Kharwars and Gonds (Majhis). In return for supplying this cloth at marriages they used to get grains, cash and at times a piece of land. Some Panikas said that in good old days cotton grew well in the slash and burn fields. With the end of the practice of shifting cultivation the availability of cotton decreased and they had to abandon cloth weaving. Majumdar (1966) mentions that *tasar* (non-mulberry silk) weaving was also practised widely by the Panka some forty-fifty years ago. But that industry had also declined. Presently some efforts are being made by the government to revive it.

Now, the Panika are cultivators of small holdings, in comparison to the Gond or Kharwar and work as agriculture labourers. Among their working population, 68.7 per cent were agriculturists, 19.7 per cent agricultural labour and the remaining 11.6 per cent depended on livestock rearing, household industry, construction work, etc. (Census 1961).

The agricultural practices of the Panika are similar to those of the Kharwar and Gond. The Baiga is called by them also for different rituals connected with agriculture. Men and women both work in agriculture but ploughing can be done only by men. Collection of minor forest produce was also undertaken to supplement their income. But this source of livelihood is gradually drying up.

In the Singrauli area, the Panika had a larger population. Their economic condition was better because land was fertile and keeping of cattle for milk was prevalent. Womenfolk used to collect fuel wood and *sal* leaves from the forest.

The Panika live in mixed villages with other tribes and castes. Their houses are *kachcha*, made of mud walls with small rooms or *kothari* and thatched roofing. Poorer persons live in huts with little accommodation. Their houses are generally huddled together because their agricultural holdings are small or they may be landless.

Open space in front of the house is used for cattle. In the Singrauli area their houses were bigger.

The Panika observe no ceremony during pregnancy. The delivery is usually conducted by an elderly Panika woman but in difficulty a Chamar *dai* is called. Sixth day and twelfth day ceremonies are observed. *Biyah* and *sagai* are the two types of marriage. They also call the Baiga for performing the *mat-korwa* ritual at marriages. Now, low Brahmin priests are called for performing rituals. Outside influence has given rise to the custom of dowry among them and the use of modern musical bands and decorations for the *barat* have started.

The Panika also have deep faith in ghosts and spirits who are propitiated on appropriate occasions with the help of an *Ojha* or *Baiga*. They observe all Hindu festivals celebrated in the area, but Holi and Dasahra are observed with great enthusiasm, when they make offerings to Dulha Deo, who is represented by a piece of stone or a mud platform. In the past the people in the area believed that the Panika had power to invoke god of rain and they were called to do so for timely monsoon.

The Panika have their traditional *birdari panchayat*, headed by a *Chaudhary*. Their big *panchayat* is at Singrauli, whreas smaller *panchayats* covering two to three villages function elsewhere. The office of its head, *Chaudhary*, is hereditary. The *panchayat* usually deals with cases of theft, illicit unions, violation of caste norms, family quarrels divorce, etc. Now its role has declined a great deal.

Among Panikas, literacy was quite low (4.9% in 1961) and female literacy was negligible. The position has now improved and boys are sent to schools, but girls' education is still not encouraged. A few young men have passed high school, intermediate or graduation levels. Some have gone into government service and have also become teachers. They have taken a lead in forming labour cooperative societies, social service organisations and in the agitational fora, specially in Kharia village and rehabilitation area. In a social organisation at Dibulganj, a Panika woman was an active worker. They have also associated themselves with the activities of the Banvasi Seva Ashram and the M.P. Lokayan and Lokhit Samiti. One of the most prominent leaders of the area, an ex-M.P., belongs to this caste.

The Lohar

The Lohar usually perform functions of both the carpenter and blacksmith in this area. They prefer to be known as Vishwakarma, instead of Lohar. In an average village only one family of Lohar is usually found whose services are taken for making and repairing of agricultural implements, bullock carts, crude wooden furniture, etc. They are listed as a Backward Caste in the State. Lohar's relations with other castes, particularly with agriculturists are based on *jajmani* or *pati* system. For making and repairing of agricultural implements they used to get foodgrains at the time of harvest and some small cash. At the time of marriage they supplied small wooden planks and wooden parrots and in return got some cash, grains and a saree. In Bijpur area an elderly informant of this caste said that about seven generations ago his ancestors had emigrated to Singrauli state from the north because artisan castes were given royal patronage as well as free land. Now, besides this occupation they have engaged themselves in cultivation and agricultural labour also. But before displacement they used to give their lands on *batai* to other castes/tribes. The demand for agricultural implements has now gone down after displacement of people and some of the Lohars have taken up the work of making furniture, doors, windows, etc.

They are Hindus and celebrate all Hindu festivals. In agriculture work, the Baiga is called to perform worship of the land since he is considered the master of land, and he is paid in cash and kind. Brahmin priests are consulted in different functions connected with life cycle ceremonies like marriage, birth, etc.

Literacy among them is not high, but they have started sending children to schools. They are quite aware of their rights as displaced families and hold important offices in the organisation called the Visthapit Yuva Sangharsh Samiti of Singrauli area.

The Teli

The Teli, a Backward Caste, are traditionally oil-pressers. In this area, besides their traditional occupation, they have taken to petty business like selling grocery minor forest produce and foodgrains. Now, they have adopted surnames like Gupta, Sahu, Sah, etc.

In the course of their business and money-lending they have come to acquire lands and now they are mostly agriculturists, as cultivators or even labourers. The lands have been grabbed mostly from their tribal and Scheduled Caste debtors. In other areas a custom of seeing a Teli early in the morning is taken as a bad omen but it is not so in this area. In Singrauli area they are found in large numbers as the ruler of Singrauli had given land and other facilities to the Teli, as an artisan group.

They have been paying some attention to the education of their children and show better literacy in comparison to other castes and tribes. Graduates and diploma holders are found among them. They have entered into government service as teachers, *lekhpal, amin,* etc. Some have become contractors with different government departments.

They observe all the Hindu festivals and also worship at the *baigadih, devsthan,* etc. and propitiate ghosts and spirits. They take the service of the Baiga while initiating agricultural operations and at the time of marriages. Brahmin priest is consulted on all occasions, viz. birth of a child, performance of marriage and death rites. A local

Chamar midwife is called for conducting delivery.

In our sample, a majority of them had medium to small land holdings and their houses were comparatively large. In some villages they were Pradhan or Up-Pradhan of Gramsabhas, which reflected their economic status, prosperity and influence.

They also had their caste or *biradari* panchayat which used to decide cases of violation of caste rules, family quarrels. But now it hardly functions.

The Biyar

The Biyar are a numerically important caste. The caste does not find a place in any of the lists (Scheduled Castes, Scheduled Tribes or Backward Castes) of U.P. In M.P. They are treated as a Scheduled Tribe. Drake-Brockman (1911) described them 'as of a aboriginal stock'. They are known as a caste of labourers and cultivators. The word *bair* means a seedbed and this may be the origin of their name as their principal occupation is rice cultivation and the construction of tanks and embankments. They are still noted for their skill in earth work and are employed generally in excavation works.

They are divided into two endogamous subdivisions. Barhaiya (from pargana Barhar, north of Son) and Dakhhinaha (southerners who live south of Son).

Their main deity is Mahadeva and Sewanriya, the deity of boundaries. Dharti Mahadeva the earthgod is also worshipped. Sewanriya's shrine is made on the boundary consisting of a mud platform under a *semal, bahera* or *pipal* tree (Mishra 1988). They have faith in ghosts and spirits and the Baiga or *Ojha* is consulted in this regard. The *devasthan, baiga-dih,* and temples of Shiva are propitiated on different occasions with offerings. They are Hindus and observe Hindu festivals.

Biyars formed a sizeable group in both Dudhi and Singrauli areas. In Singrauli they were engaged more in agriculture, as cultivator or labourer. Here, they also kept a good number of cattle for milk and *ghee* (purified butter) business. Collection of forest produce had been an additional source of income. In villages Barawani and Gharsani in the NCL and Anpara areas, Biyars are comparatively in large numbers.

Biyar *Biradari panchayat* was called *Taat* which was headed by a *Mukhiya*. It dealt with cases of theft, violation of caste rules, illicit sex relationships, family quarrels, etc. But its influence has decreased considerably.

In marriages, the Baiga is called for *matkorwa* connected with the marriage *mandap* and the Brahmin priest officiates at the actual marriage ceremony. Dowry was unknown but now it has become a must.

Biyars say that in the past their life was happy and peaceful. They had medium and small land holdings, and were engaged in cultivation and as labour, as well as collector of forest produce. Herbs and shrubs were collected and some Biyars were *vaid* treating different types of diseases. They were also traditional veterinary healers. Now most of them have become landless and their economic base has gone, resulting into breaking down of the *pati* custom of inter-caste relationships.

Discussion

The tribal groups or 'adivasis' are readily acknowledged by the caste groups as the *mool nivasi*, original inhabitants, of the area. The area was inhospitable, hilly and covered with dense forests and the tribal groups have been moving into or out of it from the adjoining tribal districts of Bihar and Madhya Pradesh. Some of them still mention the 'oral history' or legends of their original habitats (Majumdar 1960). The migratory movements brought about mixed tribal villages in this area, unlike villages inhabited by only one or two tribal groups in the neighbouring states. The pattern of habitation however, has been that different tribal groups in the same village live in different hamlets or *tolas*. The houses were built not in clusters but scattered in the midst of their agricultural lands, which considerably hampered intra-village communication. Sometimes, even the boundaries of the village are not well defined and the tribal residential conglomerations often change due to incidence of death or disease. The tribals were practising shifting cultivation almost till the middle of this century and their tenancy or ownership over the land remained unwritten or traditional, in the absence of a survey and record of rights. This is a common feature of the land-tiller relationship in many tribal areas (Roy-Burman 1992).

The availability of agricultural lands and the forest resources has been attracting the non-tribals to this area since long. The migrants belonged to both higher and lower Hindu castes and came from the eastern districts of U.P., Bihar and M.P. (Majumdar 1960). Gradually the non-tribals created better assets for themselves, and also indulged in the exploitation of tribal population through moneylending, debt bondage and land grabbing. The traditional moneylenders in the area are still found to extend unsecured loans at an interest of ten per cent per month. This trend increased manifold after the area lost its special status as a Partially Excluded Area (Hasan 1985).

Geographically, the entire tract inhabited by the tribal and the migrant non-tribal populations can be divided into Dudhi and Singrauli areas. In Dudhi area the land was generally rocky and therefore not very fertile. In fact the area faced frequent famines till mid-century and the tribals were the worst sufferers. Such adversities compounded with the heavy influx of outsiders and later, inequities of land and forest laws, have resulted into a defeatist outlook and 'loss of nerves' among some tribals. These adverse agricultural circumstances were often remedied, to a certain extent, by the availability of minor forest produce, which supplemented their diet and also their income. During some parts of the year they got wage work in the forests and also earned through collection of lac, tendu leaf, etc. The Dudhi area was considered as a punishment posting for the government officers. Conditions in Singrauli were better. In fact it was referred to as the 'Kashmir of Mirzapur district.' The land was fertile with some facilities of irrigation. Since the area was part of a princely state the people had better access to the forests and therefore animal husbandry too was practised on a large scale. The milch-cows of this area were well known (SETU 1985). In both the areas people remained somewhat isolated till the middle of the century. Thereafter contacts with outsiders and settling down of migrants increased due to the community development and other programmes, intensive exploitation of forest resources, etc. The construction of the Rihand dam and the setting up of power and mining projects and other industries intensified the contacts manifold and almost suddenly.

The dynamics of tribe caste relations in the villages of the area indicates that even though the process of Sanskritization was patent it has not permeated deep enough to turn the tribes into castes and bring about a transformation into peasant village communities. The forces of integration are far from strong and largely hori-zontal (Majumdar 1960). Further, interrelations between castes and tribes and their hierarchical positions are subject to changes as there are no predominant castes (of course a tribe can hardly predominate in such a situation) and the alliances keep on changing for various reasons, making the levels of cohesion fluid. In the words of Majumdar (1960), 'a *modus vivendi* has to be reached by the castes and tribes'. This also renders village leadership diffused and the politics in the villages highly variable. As already described, the pattern of habitation in the area is another aspect of the tribe caste dynamics and it also plays a role in the matter of communications and village leadership.

In the area of religion and rituals a better cohesion among castes and tribes is visible as both the tribal Baiga and Brahmin have their roles. The Baiga safeguards the villages and worships at the village shrine. Festivals, both tribal and Hindu, are well participated in by both the sections. The forms of address and other practices connected with showing of respect to elders also permeates tribe-caste relationship.

Majumdar (1960 : *Jha-Tha*) developed the concept of 'fringe village' to depict the typical village community in the Dudhi area. The characteristics of a fringe village include fluid inter caste/tribe relations leading to changing influence of any caste or tribe at a given time in the absence of any dominant caste; a homogeneity or absence of any sharp difference in living standards; extensive exploitation of tribes through a symbiotic living together; and religious tolerance and acceptance among the groups. He also observes that due to the absence of any dominant caste even the weaker sections tend to be vocal and their participa-tion in developmental process could be more active than in a non-fringe village. Majumdar (1960 : 3) has depicted the status of different tribe and caste groups in the area as below :

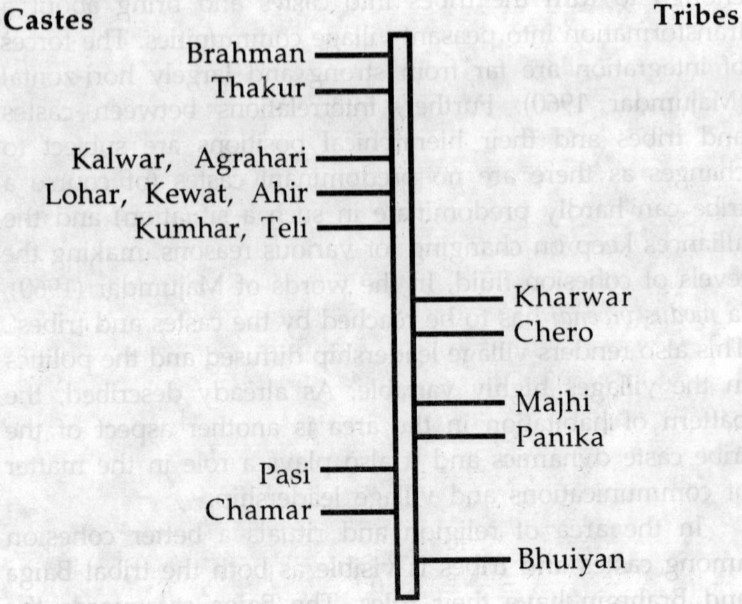

It may be added that the symbiotic living of the castes and tribes had assumed some institutionalization through the *jajmani* or *pati* relationships, a distinct feature of the village communities in India. These relations were between two groups—cultivators, and artisans and labourers. Service castes like Dhobi, Nai, Chamar and Kumhar and tribes like the Agaria and Baiga were the *pati* and the cultivators, both tribal and non-tribal, were the *jajman.* All the services rendered by the *pati* were paid through barter, in terms of a fixed quantity of grain or part cash and kind. Naturally, the *pati* were the heaviest losers when the cultivators lost their lands due to the setting up of projects as they were not entitled to any compensation for the sudden loss of their livelihood.

The above analyses pinpoints trends which have great relevance for the problem under study. The process of acquisitions of land, shifting from villages or peripheral residential areas to other places, organising the shift or even the dissemination of information related to setting up of projects, displacements, etc., and subsequently any organised attempt to resist ouster or ensuring expeditious sanctioning of claims and their payments which may include participation in judicial, quasi-legal processes, all called for three attributes, in a strong dose, for the community so affected. These were firstly, the capacity of the people to organise themselves on village community basis to take a stand on relevant issues; secondly, their ability to throw up an effective leadership to give the movement a direction and thrust and their competence in communicating meaningfully with the project, government agencies, etc., in the formal language required for such transactions on the one hand and with the community on the other; and then, of course, a network ensuring communication at not only the village but area basis among the project affected people.

The position of the Sonbhadra tribals has also to be viewed in the light of the World Bank Policy and

Guidelines relating to the relocation of displaced people in general and the tribals in particular. Cernea (1988a), Verma (1985) and Morse (1992) have discussed the definition of tribal people as spelt out by the World Bank. Briefly, the characteristics are : (a) geographically isolated or semi-isolated; (b) unacculturated or only partially acculturated into the societal norms of the dominant society; (c) nonmonetized, or only partially monetized production largely for subsistence; (d) ethnic distinctness; (e) nonliterate, without a written language; (f) linguistically distinct; (g) identifying closely with one particular territory; (h) an economic lifestyle largely dependent on the specific natural environment; (i) possessing indigenous leadership, but little or no national representation, and few, if any political rights as individuals or collectively, partly because they do not participate in the political process; and (j) having loose tenure over their traditional lands, which for the most part is not accepted by the dominant society or accommo-dated by its courts; and having weak enforcement capabilities against encroachers, even when tribal areas have been delineated.

Morse (1992 : 66), in context of the Sardar Sarovar Project, quotes the opinion expressed by the World Bank Agricultural Operations Chief that "We are not speaking of any (recognised Indian legal category such as 'scheduled tribes', but of oustees, of whatever community, *who, by nature of their physical, economic and cultural remoteness, require special treatment* if they are to regain their pre-project livelihoods", and further, "its definition tends to turn on *low degree of integration* into the large community *. . . reticence in contacts with outsiders* and possible lack of self-esteem, and other criteria as well (emphasis added). And, the data disussed in this and the previous chapters amply shows that the tribal groups in the area fit well into this paradigm.

4

DISPLACEMENT AND REHABILITATION SCENARIO

SONBHADRA has witnessed massive industrialisation from 1960 onwards, leading to displacement of several thousand families. Undoubtedly, the projects have been set up with macro developmental aims. Nonetheless all the projects have gigantic social consequences, it is not only that vast tracts of land are used or submerged for accomplishing these projects, but the people traditionally inhabiting these areas are also displaced (Bhartari and Kothari 1984). The material side of development, claimed as beneficial for all, leads to enormous socio-cultural problems, the problems arising out of displacement of people and their rehabilitation which are compounded when the displaced persons belong to the tribal and other backward communities and the area is an impoverished one.

This chapter is based on extensive field work in the area, lasting for about six months. The research methods used in the field work included a family survey based on a questionnaire, observations made by the team members during their stay in the villages/colonies surveyed, leisurely discussions with the PAPs and their leaders, collecting or upgrading ethnographic data regarding the castes and tribes in the area and discussions with some officers and representatives of the non-government organisations functioning in the area.

As stated earlier, about 50,000 persons or 10,000 families were ousted due to the setting up of six projects covered by this study. A total number of 1,038 oustee families were contacted for the survey. The families were selected on a random basis, while providing heavier representation (70%) to the tribals and Scheduled Castes, the main subject for this study. Of the remaining 30 per cent families, the backward castes and the higher castes were included for making necessary comparisons.

The family schedule was a semi-structured one and included quite a few open ended questions and questions requiring descriptive answers. Details pertaining to the demographic characteristic, material assets and land holdings before and after displacement, rehabilitation measures, compensation package, level of satisfaction, present occupations and problems faced by the oustees were collected from the selected families. The project-wise break up is mentioned in Table 4.1.

TABLE 4.1 : **Project-wise List of Families Surveyed**

Sl. No.	Name of the Project	Displacement started in the year	Number of Families surveyed
1.	Rihand Reservoir (Rihand)	1960	194
2.	Singrauli Super Thermal Power Project, Shaktinagar (Singrauli)	1977	177
3.	Anpara Thermal Power Project (Anpara)	1978	89
4.	Coal Fields—Kakri, Bina and Khadia (NCL)	1979	223
5.	Rihand Nagar Super Thermal Power Project (Bijpur)	1982	176
6.	Kanhar Irrigation Project (Kanhar)	1978	179
	Total		1038

Number of Villages/Colonies Covered

A total number of fifty-seven villages colonies were surveyed where the schedules were administered (Table 4.2). The Rihand oustees were surveyed in eleven villages/colonies, the Singrauli and Anpara oustees were covered in four villages/colonies each, the NCL oustees were covered in eighteen villages, the Bijpur oustees were taken from seven villages and the Kanhar oustees were surveyed from seventeen villages. In five out of these fifty-seven villages/colonies, oustees from more than one project have settled. They are at Khairahi re-settlement colony, Nemna and Jhilo villages, where oustees from both Rihand and Bijpur live together; whereas in Chilkadand rehabilitation colony and Chaube Paraswar village, oustees from both Singrauli and NCL live together.

Demographic Characteristics

Community-wise Distribution of Families

A majority of families in the sample comprised of the tribals (Table 4.3), which is the most significant (population-wise) group in the area. They constituted 51.9 per cent of sample families, belonging to eight tribal groups : Gond, Panika, Kharwar, Baiga, Kol, Agaria, Bhuiyar and Chero. Out of these groups, Gond, Panika and Kharwar are found in large number in the area. The Scheduled Castes comprise of 17.7 per cent families in the sample. They are: Chamar, Dharkar, Dhobi, Kori and Ghasia. Of the remaining sample 21.7 per cent of families belongs to the backward castes such as Barhi, Sonar, Teli, Lohar, Ahir, Koiri, Kahar, Kumhar, Nai, Kewat, Gosain, Kunbi, Gaderia and Muslim occupational castes. The rest 8.7 per cent belong to the other castes : Brahmins, Kayastha, Kshatriya, Bania and Biyar. Thus a total of thirty-two communities are included in the sample (which covers almost all the communities) out of which eight are tribes, five are Scheduled Castes, fourteen are backward castes and the rest five belong to other castes.

TABLE 4.2 : **Families Surveyed-Village and Project-wise**

Sl. No.	Name of the Village	Ri-hand	Sing-rauli	An-para	NCL	Bij-pur	Kan-har
1	2	3	4	5	6	7	8
1.	Khairahi (Resettlement)	19	—	—	—	1	—
2.	Liladabo	10	—	—	—	—	—
3.	Babhni	30	—	—	—	—	—
4.	Sirsoti	22	—	—	—	—	—
5.	Mahrikala	29	—	—	—	—	—
6.	Jaraha	13	—	—	—	—	—
7.	Nemna	5	—	—	—	15	—
8.	Ras Pahari	2	—	—	—	—	—
9.	Kundadih	2	—	—	—	—	—
10.	Jhilo	32	—	—	—	1	—
11.	Sodhau	30	—	—	—	—	—
12.	Chilkadand	—	145	—	36	—	—
13.	Chaube Paraswar	—	3	—	1	—	—
14.	Babu Paraswar	—	3	—	—	—	—
15.	Raja Paraswar	—	26	—	—	—	—
16.	Anpara	—	12	—	—	—	—
17.	Dibulganj	—	53	—	—	—	—
18.	Audi	—	6	—	—	—	—
19.	Kakri	—	9	—	—	—	—
20.	Bansi	—	9	—	—	—	—
21.	Ambedkar Nagar	—	—	—	32	—	—
22.	Punarvas-3	—	—	—	1	—	—
23.	Khadia	—	—	—	24	—	—
24.	Koharaulia	—	—	—	16	—	—
25.	Kohraul	—	—	—	8	—	—
26.	Misra	—	—	—	15	—	—
27.	Bhairwa	—	—	—	2	—	—
28.	Yogi Chaura	—	—	—	4	—	—

(Contd.)

TABLE 4.2 : ***(Contd.)***

1.	2.	3.	4.	5.	6.	7.	8.
29.	Marrak	—	—	—	16	—	—
30.	Rakhi Bandhi	—	—	—	3	—	—
31.	Gharsani	—	—	—	22	—	—
32.	Chanduwar	—	—	—	14	—	—
33.	Jawahar Nagar	—	—	—	5	—	—
34.	Barwani	—	—	—	9	—	—
35.	Bansi (Bina)	—	—	—	12	—	—
36.	Khokhra	—	—	—	3	—	—
37.	Dodhar	—	—	—	—	47	—
38.	Aghaura	—	—	—	—	20	—
39.	Metihani	—	—	—	1	1	—
40.	Bijpur	—	—	—	—	91	—
41.	Gohra	—	—	—	—	—	10
42.	Lambi	—	—	—	—	—	17
43.	Korchhi	—	—	—	—	—	32
44.	Randah Tola	—	—	—	—	—	15
45.	Ghusur	—	—	—	—	—	13
46.	Karchhatola	—	—	—	—	—	1
47.	Sugwa Mand	—	—	—	—	—	15
48.	Bagahdu	—	—	—	—	—	4
49.	Milsikala	—	—	—	—	—	1
50.	Amwar	—	—	—	—	—	13
51.	Jamuwani	—	—	—	—	—	1
52.	Barkhoda	—	—	—	—	—	10
53.	Kudari	—	—	—	—	—	1
54.	Sundari	—	—	—	—	—	35
55.	Nandhiha	—	—	—	—	—	1
56.	Barkhora	—	—	—	—	—	1
57.	Kuchchri	—	—	—	—	—	9
	Total	174	177	89	223	176	179

TABLE 4.3 : **Community-wise Distribution of Families (Project-wise)**

Sl. No.	Caste		Rihand	Singrauli	Anpara	NCP	Bijpur	Kanhar	Total
1	2		3	4	5	6	7	8	9
1.	Gond	T	61(31.4)	—	02(02.3)	02(01.0)	51(29.0)	14(07.8)	130(12.5)
2.	Panika	T	36(18.6)	12(06.8)	15(16.8)	20(09.0)	36(20.5)	01(00.6)	120(11.6)
3.	Kharwar	T	27(13.9)	—	43(48.3)	12(05.4)	01(00.6)	54(30.2)	137(13.2)
4.	Baiga	T	35(18.0)	08(04.5)	—	06(02.7)	29(16.5)	—	78(07.5)
5.	Kol	T	06(03.1)	11(06.2)	—	07(03.1)	—	—	24(02.3)
6.	Agaria	T	03(01.6)	—	—	—	—	—	03(00.3)
7.	Bhuiyar	T	—	—	—	—	—	39(21.8)	39(03.9)
8.	Chero	T	—	—	—	—	—	07(03.9)	07(00.7)
9.	Chamar	SC	04(02.1)	38(21.4)	16(18.0)	56(25.1)	08(04.5)	12(06.7)	134(12.9)
10.	Dharkar	SC	—	05(02.8)	—	—	06(03.4)	—	11(01.0)
11.	Dhobi	SC	06(03.1)	10(05.6)	—	02(01.0)	—	02(01.1)	20(01.9)
12.	Kori	SC	—	12(06.8)	—	—	—	—	12(01.2)
13.	Ghasia	SC	—	—	—	—	—	07(03.9)	07(00.7)
14.	Barhi	BC	—	—	—	—	05(02.8)	—	05(00.5)
15.	Sonar	BC	—	03(01.7)	—	—	—	—	03(00.3)
16.	Teli	BC	—	22(12.4)	—	21(09.4)	17(09.7)	—	60(05.8)
17.	Lohar	BC	01(00.5)	12(06.8)	01(01.1)	09(04.0)	03(01.7)	03(01.7)	29(02.8)

18.	Ahir	BC	—	07(04.0)	05(05.6)	06(02.7)	02(01.1)	18(10.0)	38(03.7)
19.	Koiri	BC	—	—	01(01.1)	11(04.9)	—	—	12(01.2)
20.	Kahar	BC	—	06(03.4)	—	05(02.2)	—	01(00.6)	12(01.2)
21.	Kumhar	BC	—	—	—	01(00.5)	—	07(03.9)	08(00.8)
22.	Nai	BC	—	06(03.4)	01(01.1)	05(02.2)	01(01.1)	01(00.6)	14(01.3)
23.	Kewat	BC	—	02(01.1)	—	03(01.3)	05(02.8)	—	10(00.9)
24.	Gosain	BC	—	—	—	—	—	02(01.1)	02(00.2)
25.	Muslim	BC	—	02(01.1)	02(02.3)	08(03.6)	—	08(04.4)	20(01.9)
26.	Kunbi	BC	—	03(01.7)	—	06(02.7)	—	—	09(00.8)
27.	Gaderia	BC	—	—	—	—	03(01.7)	—	03(00.3)
28.	Kayastha	O	—	02(01.1)	—	—	—	—	02(00.2)
29.	Brahmin	O	—	07(04.0)	—	05(02.2)	05(02.8)	—	17(01.6)
30.	Bania	O	01(00.5)	04(02.3)	02(02.3)	01(00.5)	03(01.7)	03(01.7)	14(01.3)
31.	Biyar	O	14(07.2)	01(01.1)	01(01.1)	37(16.5)	01(00.6)	—	54(05.2)
32.	Kshatriya	O	—	04(02.3)	—	—	—	—	04(00.4)
	Total		174	177	89	223	176	179	1038

Note : Figures in the parenthesis indicate column percentage.

T—Tribal, SC—Scheduled Caste, BC—Backward Caste and O—Other Castes.

Family Size

The size of the families in the area varied from small families having five members or less to very large families having more than twenty-five members (Table 4.4). A majority of families (42.4%) are of medium size (6-10 members). Over all, 74.3 per cent of families have 1 to 10 members. This trend is found in all the rehabilitation colonies/villages of all projects except Kanhar where more than 40 per cent families are large sized, i.e. 10+ members. The reason for this pattern is that in Kanhar the people have yet to be displaced and they are continuing with their old pattern of life.

Age Group of the Informants

The age of the informants varied between 21 years to more than 61 years. In some cases the informants were 80 years old. It may be seen from Table 4.5, that the informants belonged almost evenly to all the age groups, i.e. 18 to 22 per cent, except for the oldest age group of 61 years and above. The oldest age group constituted 13.9 per cent in the sample. However, in case of Rihand oustees, only 3 per cent belonged to the youngest age group (21 to 30) since Rihand displacement occurred long back. Thus the age group of the informants provided representation of all generations.

Literacy

Most of the oustees (61 per cent) are illiterates (Table 4.6). The Anpara oustees are the most literate (47.2 per cent) whereas the Rihand oustees are the least literate (32 per cent).

Displacement and Rehabilitation

Prior Notice to the Oustees

In case of Rihand oustees, most of them do not remember about the notice. Only eight respondents informed that a

TABLE 4.4 : **Family Size (Project-Wise)**

Sl. No.	No. of Members	Rihand	Singrauli	Anpara	NCL	Bijpur	Kanhar	Total
1.	01-05	47(24.2)	59(33.3)	35(39.3)	66(29.6)	86(48.9)	38(21.2)	331(31.9)
2.	06-10	85(43.8)	84(47.5)	38(42.7)	100(44.9)	66(37.5)	67(37.4)	440(42.4)
3.	11-15	37(19.1)	22(12.4)	6(6.7)	33(14.8)	12(6.8)	41(22.9)	151(14.5)
4.	16-20	17(08.7)	4(02.3)	5(05.6)	15(06.7)	9(05.1)	21(11.7)	71(06.8)
5.	21-25	4(02.1)	5(02.8)	3(03.4)	5(02.2)	3(01.7)	5(02.8)	25(02.4)
6.	26 & above	4(02.1)	3(01.7)	2(02.3)	4(01.8)	—	7(04.0)	20(02.0)
	Total	194(100)	177(100)	89(100)	223(100)	176(100)	179(100)	1038(100)

Note : Figures in the parenthesis indicate column percentage.

TABLE 4.5 : **Age Group of the Informants (Project-Wise)**

Sl. No.	Age group in years	Rihand	Singrauli	Anpara	NCL	Bijpur	Kanhar	Total
1.	21-30	6(03.0)	59(33.3)	15(16.8)	86(38.6)	42(23.8)	19(10.6)	227(21.9)
2.	31-40	50(25.8)	52(29.4)	18(20.2)	54(24.2)	51(29.0)	37(20.7)	262(25.2)
3.	41-50	50(25.8)	24(13.6)	25(28.1)	44(19.7)	39(22.2)	38(21.2)	220(21.2)
4.	51-60	49(25.3)	29(16.4)	20(22.5)	26(11.7)	22(12.5)	39(21.8)	185(17.8)
5.	61 & above	39(20.1)	13(07.3)	11(12.4)	13(05.8)	22(12.5)	46(25.7)	144(13.9)
	Total	194(100)	177(100)	89(100)	223(100)	176(100)	179(100)	1038(100)

Note : Figures in the parenthesis indicate column percentage.

TABLE 4.6 : **Literacy in the Area (Project-wise)**

Sl. No.	Name of the Project	Literate	Illiterate	Total
1.	Rihand	62 (32.0)	132 (68.0)	194
2.	Singrauli	68 (38.0)	109 (62.0)	177
3.	Anpara	42 (47.2)	47 (52.8)	89
4.	NCL	101 (45.3)	122 (54.7)	223
5.	Bijpur	71 (40.3)	105 (59.7)	176
6.	Kanhar	66 (36.9)	113 (63.1)	179
	Total	410 (39.0)	628 (61.0)	1038

notice of 16 to 30 days was given to vacate the area. The Singrauli oustees said that they were given a time period of 15 days to one month to vacate. Among the NCL oustees, nearly 20 per cent had no knowledge about it, whereas the rest stated that they were given 15 to 30 days notice to vacate. At Bijpur, 40 per cent oustees were not aware about any notice and the rest were given 15 to 30 days time. At Kanhar, notice has been already served and displacement is yet to take place.

Land Holding

The oustees have been badly affected because of the loss of agricultural land due to displacement. Only at Rihand land for land was the rule for rehabilitation and the Rihand oustees got land as compensation. However, some of the Rihand oustees have faced multiple displacement. Before displacements. 155 out of 194 Rihand oustees had land holdings and now 137 respondents possess some agricultural land (Table 4.7). In the remaining four projects, as many as 70 per cent possessed agricultural land before displacement. At

TABLE 4.7 : **Family-wise Land Holding before Displacement and at present (Project-wise)**

Sl. No.	Land in bigha *	Number of Families											
		Rihand		Singrauli		Anpara		NCL		Bijpur		Total	
		Before	Present	Before	Present	Before	Present	Before	Present	Before	Present	Before	Present
1.	Nil	39	38	40	140	12	72	83	217	63	132	237	599
2.	01-10	107	136	103	24	58	9	103	5	92	38	463	212
3.	11-20	28	1	14	nil	9	nil	14	nil	11	6	76	7
4.	21-30	9	nil	3	nil	3	nil	2	1	7	nil	24	1
5.	31-40	5	nil	3	nil	nil	nil	11	nil	—	nil	19	nil
6.	41 and above	2	nil	2	nil	nil	nil	—	nil	3	nil	7	nil
7.	No reply	4	19	12	13	7	8	10	nil	—	nil	33	40

* This is *pucca* bigha = 0.57 acre or 0.24 ha.

present only 16 per cent possess land. This shows the change in the bases of economy in the area. Once the people solely depended on agriculture and after displacement they have to rely on all other possible avenues for work, other than agriculture. The land data pertaining to Kanhar, where no displacements have been mde as yet, show that out of 179 families in the sample, 91 have 1 to 10 bigha, 26 have 11 to 20 bigha, 24 have 21 to 30 bigha and the rest do not have any law.

Animals and Birds before Displacement and at Present

The animal and bird assets are important for the rural and tribal people. Among animals, milch cattle, bullocks, goats are important besides poultry birds. In most of the cases, people have lost their livestock (Table 4.8). Data for Kanhar pertains to the present position, whereas, in other five projects, it shows that before displacement a majority (69 per cent) possessed cows and buffaloes and at present only 49 per cent have got them. As many as 72 per cent had bullocks and now only 37 per cent possess bullocks. This reduction can be directly ascribed to loss of agricultural land. Regarding possession of goats, in four projects (Rihand, Singrauli, Anpara and NCL), 38 per cent had goats before displacement and at present only 28 per cent possess goats. Data available for poultry birds from two projects (Rihand and NCL) shows that only a few family possess them.

Income

Only 10.4 per cent oustees have regular employment (Table 4.9). All the rest depend on casual employment for their living. Among Rihand oustees, only two persons are on regular pay roll; 42 each are on regular employment at Singrauli and Bijpur; whereas at NCL, 23 are on regular jobs and at Kanhar just four persons are having regular jobs. Most of the persons (65 out of 113) on regular jobs received a monthly income between

TABLE 4.8 : Family-wise Number of Animals/Birds before Displacement and at present

Sl. No.	Animal/Birds	Number of Families													
		Rihand		Singrauli		Anpara		NCL		Bijpur		Kanhar		Total	
		Before	Present	Before	Present	Before	Present	Before	Present	Before	Present	Before	Present	Before	Present
1.	Cow & buffaloes :														
	Nil	57	75	60	113	16	39	63	122	70	89	—	56	266	494
	1 to 10	88	119	88	63	43	50	125	98	64	84	—	122	408	536
	11 & above	49	nil	29	1	30	nil	35	3	42	3	—	1	185	8
2.	Bullocks :														
	Nil	44	49	61	167	14	44	60	174	58	106	—	23	237	563
	1 to 10	148	102	115	10	74	45	159	49	116	70	—	156	612	432
	11 & above	2	43	1	nil	1	nil	4	nil	2	nil	—	nil	10	43
3.	Goat :														
	Nil	103	90	125	161	46	64	150	171	—	—	—	—	424	486
	1 to 10	67	98	39	15	31	25	53	49	—	—	—	—	190	187
	11 & above	24	6	13	1	12	nil	20	3	—	—	—	—	69	10
4.	Birds :														
	Nil	145	115	—	—	—	—	203	223	—	—	—	—	348	338
	1 to 10	45	74	—	—	—	—	19	nil	—	—	—	—	64	74
	11 & above	4	5	—	—	—	—	1	nil	—	—	—	—	5	5

Note : — indicates data not available.

Rs. 1501 to 2000 which indicates that all of them were placed in the lowest category of positions.

TABLE 4.9 : **Average Income per month from Regular Employment (Project-wise)**

Sl. No.	Income Range (in rupees)	Number of Families						
		Ri-hand	Sing-rauli	An-para	NCL	Bij-pur	Kan-har	Total
1.	500-1000	—	—	—	—	7	—	7 (0.7)
2.	1001-1500	2	—	—	6	22	4	34 (3.3)
3.	1501-2000	—	35	—	17	13	—	65 (6.3)
4.	2001-2500	—	7	—	—	—	—	7 (0.7)
	Total	2	42	—	23	42	4	113 (10.4)
	Total Sample	194	177	89	223	176	179	1038

The average monthly income from casual labour is very poor. A staggering 65 per cent of those engaged in casual labour received less than Rs. 500 per month. Only a few (1.4 per cent) could get more than Rs. 1000 per month (Table 4.10).

The daily wage rates for casual labourers (Table 4.11) shows that a majority (70%) of labourers received less than Rs. 20 per day. The break-up shows: 14 per cent received below Rs. 10 per day, 20.2 per cent received Rs. 11 to 15 per day and 35.4 per cent received Rs. 16 to 20 per day.

The number of days in a month for which a casual labourer gets emloyment is very important for his income.

TABLE 4.10 : **Average Income per month from Casual Employment (Project-wise)**

Sl. No.	Income Range (in rupees)	Number of Families						
		Ri-hand	Sing-rauli	An-para	NCL	Bij-pur	Kan-har	Total
1.	Upto 250	87	—	29	74	—	72	262 (27.7)
2.	251-500	66	107	42	102	7	43	367 (37.4)
3.	501-750	15	20	10	10	72	20	147 (15.2)
4.	751-1000	12	0	4	5	49	10	89 (9.1)
5.	1001 & above	3	—	1	2	6	2	14 (1.4)
6.	Not specified	9	—	3	30	20	28	90 (9.2)
	Total*	192	136	89	223	154	154	969

* The total of Table 4.9 & 4.10 is more than the sample size (1038) because more than one member of a family are engaged in regular employment, casual jobs.

It has been found that as many as 43 per cent labourers get work for 16 to 20 days in a month, followed by 21.7 per cent who get 11 to 15 days work and 13 per cent get below 10 days of work in a month (Table 4.12). Most of the persons in NCL get more days of work, followed by Singrauli and Bijpur.

TABLE 4.11 : **Daily Wage Rate for Casual Employment (Project-wise)**

Sl. No.	Wage Rate (in rupees)	Number of Families						
		Ri-hand	Sing-rauli	An-para	NCL	Bij-pur	Kan-har	Total
1.	Upto 10	13	nil	3	nil	nil	115	131 (14.0)
2.	11-15	93	nil	7	26	60	9	195 (20.2)
3.	16-20	65	60	73	98	40	7	343 (35.4)
4.	21-25	5	50	6	63	13	7	144 (14.4)
5.	26-30	3	10	nil	3	10	nil	26 (2.6)
6.	31-35	1	16	nil	1	6	nil	24 (2.5)
7.	36-40	1	nil	nill	2	4	nil	7 (0.7)
8.	Not specified	11	nil	nil	30	21	37	99 (10.2)
	Total	192	136	89	223	154	175	969

Community-wise Employment Position

The oustees are engaged in various types of jobs such as casual labourers, regular employees of some organisation or self employed in their shops. Among Rihand oustees, most of the people are engaged in agricultural labour and labour work with the contractors (Table 4.13). Only two persons are employed on a regular basis in NTPC Bijpur. Among the tribals some families have taken up work of masonry at Renukoot. Among Singrauli oustees, forty two families derive their livelihood from employment on

TABLE 4.12: **Number of Days Employed as Casual Labourer in a Month (Project-wise)**

Sl. No.	Number of days	Number of Families						
		Rihand	Singrauli	Anpara	NCL	Bijpur	Kanhar	Total
1.	Upto 10	60	nil	48	10	9	nil	127 (13.0)
2.	11 to 15	66	28	21	8	36	45	204 (21.7)
3.	16 to 20	36	87	11	157	66	61	418 (43.0)
4.	21 to 25	10	16	5	11	20	27	89 (9.0)
5.	26 to 30	9	5	4	7	3	9	37 (3.6)
6.	Not specified	11	nil	nil	30	20	33	94 (9.7)
	Total	192	136	89	223	154	175	969

TABLE 4.13 : **Community-wise Nature of Employment at Rihand**

Sl. No.	Community	Num- of Families	Casual							Regular
			No	Agri. labour	Labour with contr.	Other+ contr. labour	Pvt. labour	Home Guard	Other	
1.	Gond	61	2	08	30	15	3	—	1	2
2.	Panika	36	1	10	15	06	4	—	—	—
3.	Baiga	35	1	14	05	14	1	—	—	—
4.	Kharwar	27	1	02	21	03	—	1	—	—
5.	Kol	06	1	02	3	—	—	—	—	—
6.	Agaria	03	—	—	3	—	—	—	—	—
7.	Chamar	04	—	1	—	03	—	—	—	—
8.	Dhobi	06	—	5	—	01	—	—	—	—
9.	Lohar	01	—	—	—	—	1	—	—	—
10.	Bania	01	—	—	1	—	—	—	—	—
11.	Biyar	14	—	1	11	1	1	—	—	—
	Total	194	5	43	89	43	10	1	1	2

a regular basis in NTPC (37) and NCL (5) whereas 135 families earn their living by pursuing casual type of employment mostly labour (130), service (7) and shop (5) (Table 4.14). The tribals such as the Baiga, Dharkar, Kol did not get any employment in NTPC or NCL. However, among the Panika, 3 got employment in NTPC.

TABLE 4.14 : **Community-wise Nature of Employment at Singrauli**

Sl. No.	Community	Number of Families	Casual employment			Regular Employment	
			Labour	Service	Shop	NTPC	NCL
1.	Ahir	07	4	2	—	1	—
2.	Biyar	01	1	—	—	—	—
3.	Baiga	08	8	—	—	—	—
4.	Brahmin	07	5	1	—	1	—
5.	Bania	04	2	—	—	2	—
6.	Chamar	38	30	—	—	6	2
7.	Dhobi	10	5	—	3	2	—
8.	Dharkar	05	5	—	—	—	—
9.	Kori	12	6	1	1	3	1
10.	Kohar	06	3	—	—	3	—
11.	Kol	11	11	—	—	—	—
12.	Kunbi	03	—	—	—	3	—
13.	Kewat	02	2	—	—	—	—
14.	Lohar	12	8	1	—	2	1
15.	Kayastha	02	—	1	—	1	—
16.	Muslim	02	2	—	—	—	—
17.	Nai	06	4	—	—	2	—
18.	Panika	12	9	—	—	3	—
19.	Kshatriya	04	2	1	—	—	1
20.	Sonar	03	2	—	—	1	—
21.	Teli	22	15	—	1	6	—
	Total	177	124	7	5	37	5

The UPSEB, which runs the Anpara project, issued instructions to the project authorities in June 1979 to provide work to one person per affected family, if the land lost by the family is fifty per cent or more of its total holding. The families losing more than fifty per cent of their land would be considered on priority basis. According to the project authorities, 261 persons were given jobs in the project. However, in our sample not a single oustee had a regular job in the project (Table 4.15). Most of the families depend upon casual labour only.

TABLE 4.15 : **Community-wise Nature of Employment at Anpara**

Sl. No.	Community	Number of Families	Casual				Regular
			None	Labour	Forest contractors	Others	
1.	Ahir	05	—	4	—	1	—
2.	Biyar	01	—	1	—	—	—
3.	Chamar	16	—	16	—	—	—
4.	Gond	02	—	2	—	—	—
5.	Bania	02	—	2	—	—	—
6.	Koiri	01	—	1	—	—	—
7.	Kharwar	43	2	39	1	1	—
8.	Lohar	01	—	1	—	—	—
9.	Muslim	02	—	1	—	1	—
10.	Nai	01	—	1	—	—	—
11.	Panika	15	—	15	—	—	—
	Total	89	2	83	1	3	nil

In NCL 202 families depend on casual labour either with contractors or others : 17 families belonging to Ahir (1), Chamar (10), Kharwar (1), Lohar (1), Muslim (1) Kunbi (1) and Teli (2) castes have thir bread-winners in different types of services; One Chamar informant is a driver, one Muslim has a shop and one Panika and one Teli are engaged in social service (Table 4.16). Only twenty-three informants are in regular employment, twelve are working in NCL and eleven in NTPC.

TABLE 4.16 : **Community-wise Nature of Employment at NCL**

Sl. No.	Community	Number of Families	Casual					Regular	
			Driver	Labour	Service	Shop	Social service	NCL	NTPC
1.	Ahir	06	—	5	1	—	—	—	—
2.	Biyar	37	—	37	—	—	—	—	—
3.	Bania	01	—	1	—	—	—	—	—
4.	Baiga	06	—	6	—	—	—	—	—
5.	Brahmin	05	—	5	—	—	—	1	—
6.	Chamar	56	1	45	10	—	—	7	4
7.	Dhobi	02	—	2	—	—	—	—	—
8.	Gond	02	—	2	—	—	—	—	—
9.	Koiri	11	—	11	—	—	—	—	—
10.	Kahar	05	—	5	—	—	—	—	—
11.	Kharwar	12	—	11	1	—	—	—	—
12.	Kumhar	01	—	1	—	—	—	—	—
13.	Kol	07	—	7	—	—	—	—	—
14.	Kunbi	06	—	5	1	—	—	—	—
15.	Kewat	03	—	3	—	—	—	—	—
16.	Lohar	09	—	8	1	—	—	—	—
17.	Muslims	08	—	6	1	1	—	—	1
18.	Nai	05	—	5	—	—	—	—	2
19.	Panika	20	—	19	—	—	1	1	—
20.	Teli	21	—	18	2	—	1	2	3
	Total	223	1	202	17	1	2	12	11

At Bijpur, forty-two families derive their livelihood from employment on a regular basis while the number of such families elsewhere is : in NTPC (27), NCL

TABLE 4.17 : **Community-wise Nature of Employment at Bijpur**

Sl. No.	Community	Number of families	Casual Employment					Regular Employment			
			Agri-culture	Labour	Animal Husb.	Service	Shop	Govt.	NTPC	NCL	Other
1.	Ahir	2	—	1	1	—	—	—	—	—	—
2.	Biyar	1	—	1	—	—	—	—	—	—	—
3.	Baiga	29	1	17	7	1	—	—	3	—	—
4.	Gond	51	3	23	3	5	—	2	10	1	4
5.	Brahmin	5	—	—	2	2	—	—	—	—	1
6.	Bania	3	—	—	—	—	2	—	—	1	—
7.	Chamar	8	—	7	—	—	—	—	1	—	—
8.	Dharkar	6	—	6	—	—	—	—	—	—	—
9.	Gaderia	2	—	2	—	—	—	—	—	—	—
10.	Kharwar	1	—	1	—	—	—	—	—	—	—
11.	Kewat	5	—	4	—	1	—	—	—	—	—
12.	Lohar	3	—	2	—	—	—	—	1	—	—
13.	Nai	1	—	—	—	1	—	—	—	—	—
14.	Panika	36	2	18	2	6	—	1	6	1	—
15.	Pal	1	—	1	—	—	—	—	—	—	—
16.	Teli	17	—	6	—	2	—	—	5	—	4
17.	Vishwakarma	5	—	3	1	—	—	—	1	—	—
	Total	176	6	92	16	18	2	3	27	3	9

(3), government departments (3) and others (9) whereas, the remaining 134 families eke out their living by pursuing casual employment mostly labour (92), service (18), animal husbandry (16), agriculture (6) and shop (2) (Table 4.17). It is worth mentioning that among tribals, only two Gonds and one Panika have got jobs in a government department, three Baiga, ten Gonds and six Panika got job in NTPC, and one Gond and one Panika got job in NCL.

At Kanhar three Ahir and one Kharwar are in regular employment in the Irrigation Department (Table 4.18). Under casual employment, one Bhuiya and one Muslim are contractors, four Bhuiya and one Muslim work with the Forest Department, one Bania and four Muslims have shops and the rest are engaged as labourers with contractors or in other types of labour work.

Compensation

Amount of Compensation Received

The oustees of various projects under study received compensation in cash in lieu of their assets. Some of the oustees (9.2 per cent) have so far received no cash compensation as reported by them (Table 4.19). A little above 18 per cent families received cash compensation below 500 rupees, and 57 per cent families received compensation ranging between 1000 rupees and 20,000 rupees. In Rihand, a majority (62.3 per cent) received below 500 rupees each. In Singrauli, 42.3 per cent received 1000 rupees to 5,000 rupees each and 38.5 per cent received more than 5000 rupees each. In case of Anpara 37 per cent received 2500 to 10000 rupees each, and in NCL about 36 per cent received the same amount each. At Bijpur, 23.3 per cent received a cash compensation of 10,000 rupees to 20,000 rupees each, closely followed by 19.3 per cent who received Rs. 5000 to Rs. 10,000 each.

TABLE 4.18 : **Community-wise Nature of Employment at Kanhar**

Sl. No.	Community	Number of families	Casual						Regular
			Not Specific	Contractors	Contractors and others	Forest	Labour	Shop	
1.	Ghasia	7	1	—	5	—	1	—	—
2.	Ahir	18	5	—	7	—	3	—	3
3.	Bhuiya	39	8	1	17	4	9	—	—
4.	Bania	3	1	—	—	—	1	1	—
5.	Chamar	12	1	—	8	—	3	—	—
6.	Dhobi	2	—	—	1	—	1	—	—
7.	Gosain	2	1	—	1	—	—	—	—
8.	Gond	14	2	—	12	—	—	—	—
9.	Kahar	1	—	—	1	—	—	—	—
10.	Baiga	7	—	—	7	—	—	—	—
11.	Kharwar	54	13	—	29	—	11	—	1
12.	Kumhar	7	1	—	1	—	5	—	—
13.	Lohar	3	—	—	3	—	—	—	—
14.	Muslim	8	—	1	—	1	2	4	—
15.	Nai	1	—	—	—	—	1	—	—
16.	Panika	1	—	—	1	—	—	—	—
	Total	179	33	2	93	5	37	5	4

TABLE 4.19 : **Amount of Compensation Received**

Sl. No.	Amount (in Rs.)	Number of Families						Total
		Rihand	Singrauli	Anpara	NCL	Bijpur	Kanhar	
1.	Nil	21 (10.8)	17 (09.6)	1 (01.1)	14 (06.3)	5 (02.9)	38 (21.2)	96 (09.2)
2.	Below 500	121 (62.3)	4 (02.3)	14 (15.7)	30 (13.5)	18 (10.2)	3 (01.7)	190 (18.3)
3.	500-1000	18 (09.3)	13 (07.3)	8 (09.0)	18 (08.1)	7 (04.0)	—	64 (5.2)
4.	1001-2500	18 (09.3)	32 (18.0)	11 (12.4)	40 (17.9)	25 (14.2)	18 (10.1)	144 (14.0)
5.	2501-5000	8 (04.1)	43 (24.3)	16 (18.0)	38 (17.0)	21 (11.9)	22 (12.3)	148 (14.3)
6.	5001-10000	5 (02.6)	27 (15.3)	17 (19.1)	42 (18.8)	39 (19.3)	31 (17.3)	156 (15.0)
7.	10001-20000	3 (01.6)	26 (14.7)	14 (15.7)	23 (10.3)	41 (23.3)	34 (19.0)	141 (13.6)
8.	20001-30000	—	8 (04.5)	3 (03.4)	8 (03.6)	12 (06.8)	14 (07.8)	45 (04.3)
9.	30001-50000	—	7 (04.0)	5 (05.6)	6 (02.7)	4 (02.3)	8 (04.5)	30 (02.9)
10.	50001 and above	—	—	—	4 (01.8)	9 (05.1)	11 (06.1)	24 (02.3)
	Total	194	177	89	223	176	179	1038

At Kanhar, 6.1 per cent oustees received more than Rs. 50,000 as cash compensation. Overall, in three projects, viz. NCL, Bijpur and Kanhar some oustee families received more than Rs. 50,000 each.

Compensation to the Rihand oustees were fixed at 30 times of the land revenue (Re. 1 per bigha) which was quite a low amount. At Singrauli and Anpara, it was Rs. 4500 per acre, which again was low compared to the land prices in the market.

Compensation Position, Community-wise

It has been found that the tribals in all projects received less compensation as compared to the other communities. At Rihand, among this group the range of compensation was upto Rs. 2500 except the Gond who got upto Rs. 20,000 (Table 4.20). These Gond families are from Sirosoti and Jheelo villages who received compensation from NTPC Bijpur, also. Thus these high figures do not reflect the compensation money received as Rihand oustees alone. In Rihand compensation for all the communities ranged below Rs. 2500. Several oustees got merely Rs. 30 to Rs. 100 which amply supports the fact that the compensation was too meagre.

At Singrauli the amount of compensation among the tribals is relatively low since no family got above Rs. 30,000 (Table 4.21). The breakup is that out of thirty-one families, two did not get any compensation, one got below Rs. 500; five got between Rs. 500 and 1000; eleven got Rs. 1000 to 2500; five each between 2500-5000 and Rs. 5000 to 10,000 and one each between Rs. 10,000 and Rs. 20,000 and Rs. 20,000 to Rs. 30,000. Amongst Scheduled Castes, the position is comparatively better since two families, got compensation between Rs. 30,000 and Rs. 50,000 (highest in this cluster). Further, out of sixty-five families, nine did not get any compensation; two got below Rs. 500; six got between Rs. 500 and 1000; nine got between Rs. 1000-2500 and twenty Rs. 2500 to 5000;

TABLE 4.20 : **Community-wise Amount of Compensation at Rihand**

Sl. No.	Community	Number of families	Amount (in Rs.)							
			Nil	Below 500	500-1000	1000-2500	2500-5000	5000-10000	10000-20000	Above 20000
1.	Gond	61	6	28	6	5	8	5	3	—
2.	Panika	36	2	21	6	7	—	—	—	—
3.	Baiga	35	8	24	1	2	—	—	—	—
4.	Kharwar	27	—	25	2	—	—	—	—	—
5.	Kol	6	2	3	1	—	—	—	—	—
6.	Agaria	3	—	3	—	—	—	—	—	—
			18	104	16	14	8	5	3	—
7.	Chamar	4	—	3	—	1	—	—	—	—
8.	Dhobi	6	1	4	1	—	—	—	—	—
			1	7	1	1	—	—	—	—
9.	Lohar	1	—	—	—	1	—	—	—	—
			—	—	—	1	—	—	—	—
10.	Bania	1	—	1	—	—	—	—	—	—
11.	Biyar	14	2	9	1	2	—	—	—	—
			2	10	1	2	—	—	—	—
	Total	194	21	121	18	18	8	5	3	—

TABLE 4.21 : **Community-wise Amount of Compensation at Singrauli**

Sl. No.	Community	Number of Families	Amount (in Rs.)									
			Nil	Below 500	500-1000	1000-2500	2500-5000	5000-10000	10000-20000	20000-30000	30000-50000	Above 50000
1.	Panika	12	2	—	—	5	2	2	1	—	—	—
2.	Kola	11	—	1	2	2	2	3	—	1	—	—
3.	Baiga	8	—	—	3	4	1	—	—	—	—	—
		31	2	1	5	11	5	5	1	1	—	—
4.	Chamar	38	2	1	5	6	15	4	2	1	2	—
5.	Kori	12	3	—	—	1	1	1	5	1	—	—
6.	Dhobi	10	3	1	1	1	1	—	2	1	—	—
7.	Dharkar	5	1	—	—	1	3	—	—	—	—	—
		65	9	2	6	9	20	5	9	3	2	—
8.	Teli	22	3	—	2	6	4	4	3	—	—	—
9.	Lohar	12	1	—	—	—	5	1	2	3	—	—
10.	Ahir	7	—	1	—	—	1	3	1	1	—	—
11.	Nai	6	—	—	—	1	1	1	2	—	1	—
12.	Kahar	6	1	—	—	—	3	—	1	—	1	—

13. Kunbi	3	—	—	—	—	—	3	—	—	—	—
14. Sonar	3	—	—	—	—	2	1	—	—	—	—
15. Kewat	2	—	—	—	1	1	—	—	—	—	—
16. Muslim	2	—	—	—	1	—	1	—	—	—	—
	63	5	1	2	9	17	14	9	4	2	—
17. Brahmin	7	1	—	—	—	1	1	4	—	—	—
18. Kshatriya	4	—	—	—	—	—	1	2	—	1	—
19. Bania	4	—	—	—	2	—	—	—	—	2	—
20. Kayastha	2	—	—	—	1	—	1	—	—	—	—
21. Biyar	1	—	—	—	—	—	—	1	—	—	—
	18	1	—	—	3	1	3	7	—	3	—
Total	177	17	4	13	32	43	27	26	8	7	—

and six got above Rs. 20,000. All the families received some compensation except one. At Singrauli, the compensation was received by forty per cent of the oustees in two to three instalments, whereas the rest got it at one time. It is interesting to note here that some of the oustees (above 13 per cent) had to bribe the officials to get the compensation released. The amount of bribe ranged between Rs. 500 and Rs. 2500.

In Anpara, among the tribal group, one Kharwar did not get any compensation; ten got below Rs. 500 (Table 4.22) and thirty-seven out of the sixty tribal families in the sample got compensation below Rs. 5000. Among Scheduled Castes (all Chamars) the position was slightly better because four got below Rs. 500; three got Rs. 500 to 1000; two Rs. 2500-5000; two between Rs. 5000-10,000 and five above Rs. 10,000. Among the Backward Castes none got below Rs. 1000; and one got Rs. 1000-2500, while the rest were all in better compensation brackets. On the whole the lowest range of compensation (below Rs. 500 and Rs. 500 to 1000) is shared by the tribal and Scheduled Caste families.

Regarding the manner of payment of compensation money, out of the eightyeight families who got it, sixty-three (70.79%) said that they had received the whole amount at one time and twenty-five (28.0%) informed that they got it in several instalments. The families removed by the railways complained of excessive delay in the payment of compensation. But the displaced families were unanimously of the view that the amount was quite inadequate as compared to the loss they were subjected to. By and large the general reactions of the oustees were: 'No land was given'; 'No jobs were given', 'No help in shifting was provided', 'Forcible eviction was made' and now 'even labour work, after losing agricultural land is difficult to get'. At NCL, eight tribal oustees out of forty-seven did not get any compensation and six got below Rs. 500 (Table 4.23). Among this group only seven

TABLE 4.22 : **Community-wise Amount of Compensation at Anpara**

Sl. No.	Community	Number of Families	Amount (in Rs.) Nil	Below 500	500-1000	1000-2500	2500-5000	5000-10000	10000-20000	20000-30000	30000-50000	Above 50000
1.	Kharwar	43	1	7	3	8	6	5	10	—	3	—
2.	Panika	15	—	3	1	2	5	3	1	—	—	—
3.	Gond	2	—	—	1	—	—	—	1	—	—	—
		60	1	10	5	10	11	8	12	—	3	—
4.	Chamar	16	—	4	3	—	2	2	2	1	2	—
		16	—	4	3	—	2	2	2	1	2	—
5.	Ahir	5	—	—	—	—	—	4	—	1	—	—
6.	Muslim	2	—	—	—	—	1	1	—	—	—	—
7.	Koiri	1	—	—	—	—	—	1	—	—	—	—
8.	Nai	1	—	—	—	1	—	—	—	—	—	—
9.	Lohar	1	—	—	—	—	—	1	—	—	—	—
		10	—	—	—	1	—	1	7	—	1	—
10.	Baniya	2	—	—	—	—	1	—	—	1	—	—
11.	Biyar	1	—	—	—	—	1	—	—	—	—	—
		3	—	—	—	—	2	—	—	1	—	—
	Total	89	1	14	8	11	16	17	14	3	5	—

TABLE 4.23 : **Community-wise Amount of Compensation at NCL**

Sl. No.	Community	Number of Families	Amount (in Rs.)									
			Nil	Below 500	500-1000	1000-2500	2500-5000	5000-10000	10000-20000	20000-30000	30000-50000	Above 50000
1.	Panika	20	1	2	1	3	5	3	3	—	1	1
2.	Kharwar	12	2	—	1	3	2	2	—	1	1	—
3.	Kol	7	2	1	1	2	1	—	—	—	—	—
4.	Baiga	6	2	3	—	1	—	—	—	—	—	—
5.	Gond	2	1	—	—	1	—	—	—	—	—	—
		47	8	6	3	10	8	5	3	1	2	1
6.	Chamar	56	1	12	3	7	9	14	8	1	1	—
7.	Dhobi	2	—	—	1	—	1	1	—	—	—	—
		58	1	12	4	7	9	15	8	1	1	—
8.	Teli	21	—	—	—	2	6	5	2	3	1	2*
9.	Koiri	11	2	—	—	2	3	2	1	1	—	—
10.	Lohar	9	—	—	1	—	3	4	—	—	1	—
11.	Muslim	8	—	1	—	1	4	—	2	—	—	—
12.	Ahir	6	—	—	—	—	1	3	2	—	—	—

13.	Kunbi	6	—	—	—	1	1	2	—	1	—	1
14.	Kahar	5	—	1	—	4	—	—	—	—	—	—
15.	Nai	5	—	—	—	—	2	1	1	1	—	—
16.	Kewat	3	—	—	2	—	1	—	—	—	—	—
17.	Kumhar	1	—	—	—	1	—	—	—	—	—	—
		75	2	2	3	11	21	17	8	6	2	3
18.	Biyar	37	3	10	8	12	—	1	2	—	1	—
19.	Brahmin	5	—	—	—	—	—	4	1	—	—	—
20.	Bania	1	—	—	—	—	—	—	1	—	—	—
		43	3	10	8	12	—	5	4	—	1	—
	Total	223	14	30	18	40	38	42	23	8	6	4

* Between Rs. 70000 to 80000 and between Rs. 80000 to 90000.

families received above Rs. 10,000. Among the fifty-eight Scheduled Caste families, only one did not get any compensation; ten families received compensation above Rs. 10000 and the rest below it. Among the Backward Castes, out of seventy-five families, only two did not get compensation; two got below Rs. 500; three got Rs. 500 to 1000; eleven got Rs. 1000 to 2500; twenty-one got Rs. 2500 to 5000; seventeen got Rs. 5000 to 10,000; and sixteen got Rs. 10,000 to 50,000.

Among other castes, out of forty-three families, three did not get compensation. In this group five families received compensation above Rs. 10,000 and the rest below it. Only sixteen families stated that they had to give bribe to the officials, ranging between Rs. 100 to Rs. 500 for getting compensation. Further, out of 209 families who had actually received compensation, 205 informed that they got it in one instalment and the rest said that they got it in more than two instalments. But, again, all contended that part of the compensation was still pending particularly that for trees, *bandis*, houses and wells.

At Bijapur, five families (four tribal and one Brahmin) did not get any compensation (Table 4.24). Among the tribals only the lowest range of compensation (below Rs. 500) was received by eight families and between Rs. 500 to 1000 by seven families. Compensation ranging between Rs. 2500 to 5000 was received by ten tribals, six Scheduled Castes, two Backward Castes and three other caste families. The highest range, above Rs. 50,000, was received by four tribals, one Scheduled Caste and four Backward Caste families. In this range two Gonds, one Teli, one Kewat got between Rs. 80,000 to Rs. 90,000.

A majority of respondents said that compensation for lands stated as forest lands and their assets over it like wells had not been paid so far and thirty-five out of 176 said that one-third of their house compensation was still pending. At Bijpur forty-three per cent oustees received the compensation in instalments whereas the rest received it in lumpsum.

At Kanhar, twenty-five tribals out of 115 did not got compensation, three got below Rs. 500; fifteen between Rs. 1000 and 2500 and eleven between Rs. 2500-5000 (Table 4.25). Among the tribals, highest amount (Rs. 80,000 to Rs. 90,000) was received by one Kharwar and one Bhuiya. Among the Scheduled Castes, out of twenty-one families, three did not get compensation; three got between Rs. 1000-2500; and eight between Rs. 2500 and 5000. Among Backward Castes, out of forty families, nine families did not get compensation; three got between Rs. 2500 and 5000; six between Rs. 5000 and 10,000; eight between Rs. 10,000-20,000; six between Rs. 20,000 and 30,000; three between Rs. 30,000-50,000; and five above Rs. 50,000. However, two Ahirs got between Rs. 80,000-90,000. Regarding the manner of payment, about sixty one per cent got in lumpsum whereas seventeen per cent got it in two to three instalments. In some cases payment of compensation is pending in the court for decision. All the respondents expressed that the rate, viz. Rs. 4500 per acre was low and hence, the amount of compensation was inadequate.

Utilisation of Compensation Amount

The data regarding the utilisation of compensation money by the oustees depicts a dismal picture of how the productive assets of the affected families were changed into liquid assets which were readily dissipated by the people whose perception of what they were doing was limited. In most of the cases the money was spent on domestic consumption, house construction and other such expenditures. At Rihand the amount of compensation was so meagre that the recipients could hardly put it to any lasting use. Among the Singrauli oustees, most utilised the money in house construction besides spending some part on domestic consumption. Among Anpara oustees, since most of them were left without any regular

TABLE 4.24 : **Community-wise Amount of Compensation at Bijpur**

Sl. No.	Community	Number of Families	Amount (in Rs.)									
			Nil	Below 500	500-1000	1000-2500	2500-5000	5000-10000	10000-20000	20000-30000	30000-50000	Above 50000
1	2	3	4	5	6	7	8	9	10	11	12	13
1.	Gond	51	—	1	4	10	3	8	19	4	—	20*
2.	Panika	36	1	14	2	4	3	5	4	3	—	—
3.	Baiga	29	3	3	1	6	4	4	6	—	—	2**
4.	Kharwar	1	—	—	—	—	—	1	—	—	—	—
		117	4	18	7	20	10	18	29	7	—	4
5.	Chamar	8	—	—	—	1	1	1	3	1	—	1**
6.	Dharkar	6	—	—	—	—	5	—	—	1	—	—
		14	—	—	—	1	6	1	3	2	—	1
7.	Teli	17	—	—	—	1	1	6	6	1	1	1*
8.	Barhai	5	—	—	—	1	—	—	1	—	3	—
9.	Kewat	5	—	—	—	—	—	2	—	—	—	3***

10.	Lohar	3	—	—	—	—	—	2	1	—	—	—
11.	Gaderia	3	—	—	—	—	—	2	—	1	—	—
12.	Ahir	2	—	—	—	1	—	1	—	—	—	—
13.	Nai	1	—	—	—	—	1	—	—	—	—	—
		36	—	—	—	3	2	13	8	2	4	4
14.	Brahmin	5	1	—	—	—	1	1	1	1	—	—
15.	Bania	3	—	—	—	1	2	—	—	—	—	—
16.	Biyar	1	—	—	—	—	—	1	—	—	—	—
		9	1	—	—	1	3	2	1	1	—	—
	Total	176	5	18	7	25	21	34	41	12	4	9

* Between Rs. 80,000 to 90,000

** Between Rs. 50,000 to 60,000.

*** 1 between Rs. 80,000-90,000; 1 between Rs. 70,000-80,000;
1 between Rs. 50,000-60,000.

TABLE 4.25 : **Community-wise Amount of Compensation at Kanhar**

Sl. No.	Community	Number of Families	Amount (in Rs.)									
			Nil	Below 500	500-1000	1000-2500	2500-5000	5000-10000	10000-20000	20000-30000	30000-50000	Above 50000
1.	Kharwar	54	4	3	—	7	6	9	12	5	4	4
2.	Bhuiyar	39	9	—	—	4	3	10	10	1	1	1
3.	Gond	14	9	—	—	2	1	2	—	—	—	—
4.	Baiga	7	2	—	—	2	1	—	—	—	—	—
5.	Panika	1	1	—	—	—	—	—	—	—	—	—
		115	25	3	—	15	11	23	22	6	5	5
6.	Chamar	12	3	—	—	1	4	1	1	2	—	—
7.	Ghasia	7	—	—	—	2	3	1	1	—	—	—
8.	Dhobi	2	—	—	—	—	1	—	1	—	—	—
		21	3	—	—	3	8	2	3	2	—	—
9.	Ahir	18	2	—	—	—	—	2	7	3	—	4

10.	Kumhar	7	2	—	—	—	1	2	1	1	—	—
11.	Lohar	3	—	—	—	—	1	1	—	1	—	—
11.	Gosain	2	—	—	—	—	1	—	—	—	1	—
13.	Nai	1	—	—	—	—	—	—	—	—	—	1
14.	Kahar	1	—	—	—	—	—	—	1	—	—	—
15.	Muslim	8	5	—	—	—	—	—	—	1	2	—
		40	9	—	—	—	3	6	8	6	3	5
16.	Bania	3	1	—	—	—	—	—	1	—	—	1
		3	1	—	—	—	—	—	1	—	—	1
	Total	179	38	3	—	18	22	31	34	14	8	11

source of income, they have spent it on domestic consumption. One oustee reported that he spent the money on the marriage of his daughter.

Among NCL projects affected families the amount of compensation was utilised to meet the daily necessities, i.e. household consumption by 160 families; only thirty-eight persons invested in house construction; six in performance of marriage and two in casual investments. Thus, household consumption accounted for an overwhelming utilisation of compensation in the face of no regular employment and sudden loss of agricultural lands and income.

At Bijpur a majority of families (126-71.59%) spent compensation amount on household consumption followed by construction of houses by thirty-nine families (22.16%), one family each on land purchase, marriage and shop, and two on digging of wells. The remaining five families could not specify clearly how they had used the money.

At Kanhar, seventy-five oustees who got below Rs. 10,000 stated that their money was utilised on household consumption and the remaining, all above the range of Rs. 10,000, said that besides household consumption they spent in expanding the house (which they would surely lose when the project is completed), purchase of land, marriage of daughters, repayment of debts and setting up of shops.

Allotment of House Plots

At Rihand and Kanhar house-plots were not allotted to the oustees. In the four other projects, where provision of a developed house-plot to each oustee family was the main plank of rehabilitation, no less than 35.3 per cent of such families did not get any plot. Of the remaining, 60.3 per cent families (Table 4.26) got one plot each, 3.9 per cent got two plots each and 0.5 per cent got three plots each. The size of plots differs in case of different projects. At Singrauli the plots were of 1500 sq. ft. (50′ □ 30′), at

Anpara and NCL they were of two sizes 1500 sq. fit. (50′   30′) and 2400 sq. ft. (60′ □ 40′); whereas at Bijpur the plots were of 2400 sq. ft. (60′ □ 40′).

TABLE 4.26 : **Allotment of House Plots to Families (Project-wise)**

Sl. No.	Number of Plots	Number of Families				
		Singrauli	Anpara	NCL	Bijpur	Total
1.	Nil	46 (26.0)	23 (25.8)	130 (58.3)	36 (20.5)	235 (35.3)
2.	1	177 (66.0)	66 (74.2)	83 (37.2)	135 (76.7)	401 (60.3)
3.	2	13 (7.3)	—	8 (3.6)	5 (2.8)	26 (3.9)
4.	3	1 (0.7)	—	2 (0.9)	—	3 (0.5)
	Total	177	89	223	176	665

The position in respect of the surveyed families clearly brings out that even the allotment of housing plots which was the minimal rehabilitation requirement has been substantially deficient. Further, large number of plots allotted were seen to be still lying vacant because the PAPs did not find these suitable for construction. Either the land was rocky and difficult to build upon or it was a low lying area. Infrastructural facilities for the colonies had not been developed even decades after displacements. The next chapter deals with this situation.

Other Development Programmes

In the foregoing paragraphs the rehabilitation aid

extended by the project authorities has been discussed. Broadly speaking, the authorities proved rather unhelpful except for the persons who were provided regular employment. Now, in this context the role of the State Government has also to be discussed. The government is the most important agency today for development measures on a broad spectrum. The main emphasis on this development programme is on providing employment, subsidiary or main, improvement in the traditional methods of economic activities and skill-development assistance for taking up new economic activities. The area has been a drought prone one and the soil in most cases is rocky, unirrigated and suitable only for millet and other minor food crops. Even this reasource base of the PAPs was lost in the process of the setting up of the projects. The government departments concerned with development claim to be implementing, on a substantial scale, schemes for improving soil, irrigation, providing employment as labourers under Jawahar Rojgar Yojana, drought prone area programme and a variety of schemes included under the IRDP umbrella to enable agriculturists to divert to secondary or tertiary economic activitieis. In addition there has been a special programme for the Scheduled Castes called the Special Component Plan (SCP). The main thrust of this programme is on supplementing the assistance available under the IRDP for taking up subsidiary economic activities with subsidies, reduced interest rates (DRI) and also creating marketable skills through training.

The development arm of the government with such a plethora of schemes could have been entrusted the task of providing wide and sustained support for rehabilitating the economy of PAPs on a large scale. A special role could have been expected through the SCP which had placed particuler emphasis on blocks having twenty per cent plus Scheduled Caste population (U.P. 1989). In the Sonbhadra district all the blocks fell in this category and villages having a large Scheduled Caste population were also substantial. The State Government had right from the beginning of the SCP identified such villages as a vital part of their development strategy. Instructions had also been issued that the villages with high Scheduled Caste population should be given the first priority in providing common amenities like drinking water, dispensaries, schools, etc., and all such facilities should be located in that part of the village which was inhabited by the Scheduled Castes.

TABLE 4.27 : **Number of Beneficiaries under Government Schemes**

Sl. No.	The Schemes	Number of Families						
		Ri-hand	Sing-rauli	An-para	NCL	Bij-pur	Kan-har	Total
1.	Milch catte	19	—	4	2	1	20	46
2.	Shop	2	4	1	1	—	3	11
3.	Housing	2	—	1	2	1	1	7
4.	Pumpsets	2	—	1	—	—	5	8
5.	Bullock	1	—	—	—	—	3	4
6.	Readymade garments	1	—	—	—	—	1	2
7.	Dug well	2	—	—	—	—	—	2
8.	Piggery	—	—	—	—	—	—	4
9.	Fertilizer	1	—	1	—	—	4	6
10.	Not specified	1	1	1	—	—	5	8
	Total	31	5	9	5	2	46	98

In this context the families surveyed were specifically asked to give details of the benefits, if any, received by them through the development schemes launched by the government departments. Significantly, the picture that emerged shows this work in a poor light. Only 9.4 per cent (98 out of 1038) of the oustees reported having taken benefit of any such scheme. The schemes availed were purchase of milch cattle or bullock, supply of fertilizers and seeds, installing pump sets and digging wells for irrigation, piggery, setting up shops, units of ready-made garments and housing facilities (Table 4.27). Almost half (46 out of 98) had benefited from the milch cattle scheme, followed by eleven oustees who got assistance for opening shops, seven persons got assistance for housing, eight got for pumpsets, six for fertilizers and four each got it for bullocks and piggery and two each obtained it for ready-made garments and well. More persons from Rihand (31 out of 98) and Kanhar (46 out of 98) could get the loans and subsidy mainly because they are still agriculturists, whereas only two persons from Bijpur, five each from the NCL region and Singrauli and nine from Anpara received assistance. In Singrauli, they got it mostly for shops. Thus, the benefits flowing from the entire range of development programmes to the worst hit oustees were negligible.

5

REHABILITATION COLONIES AND VILLAGES

IN the earlier chapter details of the fifty-seven villages/ colonies to which the surveyed families belonged have been given. In five villages/colonies oustees from more than one project were found to have been settled. These colonies were Khairahi Colony, Nemna and Jhilo villages where oustees from both Rihand and Bijpur live together, and Chilkadand Colony and Chaube Paraswar village where oustees from Singrauli and NCL were living. The study team while canvassing the family schedules also collected details of the villages/colonies involved through a simple colony/village schedule and in the course of their stay in the villages/colonies they recorded first hand information relating to the conditions prevailing there, views of the inhabitants and information regarding infrastructural facilities provided in the colonies or in the original villages by the project authorities as also the government agencies like panchayats, departments, etc. A brief note on each of the colonies/villages and the observations made by the residents themselves have been discussed here.

Conditions in Colonies/Villages

The project authorities have established rehabilitation

colonies/villages for the oustees. Brief notes on each of the colonies/villages follow, covering particularly the prevailing conditions in them and the problems faced by the inhabitants as observed by the survey teams and voiced by the people.

(a) Rihand

The district faced its first major wave of displacement due to the Rihand dam. The people living in the villages to be submerged when asked to vacate their abode did not pay any heed because sinking of their villages was beyond their imagination. However, the administration was repeatedly announcing through village pradhans, local leaders and revenue staff that the catchment area must be evacuated and many families ultimately waded through water and their belongings were removed by boats. The fleeing of affected population was chaotic as no resettlement or rehabilitation plans had been prepared. A large number of families settled down through their own efforts on the periphery of the reservoir and quite a good number had to travel long distances for safer shelter. Elderly people said that the government allowed them to settle according to their wish and convenience wherever they could find place.

Land was made available to the oustees by clearing forests. The cultivators were provided land in the range of 8-10 bighas and 3¼ bighas were given to artisans and landless families. People who settled on the eastern and western flanks of the reservoir had to face further displacements on account of the subsequent industrialisation in this area.

Though forest lands were assigned to the displaced families in pursuance of a government decision, the cultivators were generally not given the *pattas*. These cultivators laboured hard in removing *khoont* (tree trunks), stone boulders and levelling their lands to make them cultivable. Now after a passage of more than two decades the lands are yielding fairly good crops. But the rehabilitated are facing problems presently on account of the survey agency operating in the area for updating the land records. As the tribals and Scheduled Castes are illiterate and ignorant unscrupulous elements are trying to grab their lands. Many cultivators have no *pattas* for the allotted land and influential people try to get such lands entered in their names in the land records for instance :

(a) A Panika informed that after Rihand displacement he settled in Tola Dopiha of village Mehrikalan in 1961. He cleared the forest and reclaimed ten bighas of land for cultivation and this is the only source of livelihood for his family. But a big cultivator got this land entered in his name by the survey agency. The Panika has approached the authorities but no attention is being paid to his genuine demand.

(b) A Dharkar of Babhani village got about five bighas of land under rehabilitation and also got *patta* of another 7½ bighas of Gaon Sabha land. He has been paying Rs. 6.60 as revenue regularly and has its receipt of March 1990. Some influential persons have got most of his land entered in their names. Though a case has been filed by him he is not sure of its outcome and is very much disturbed.

The oustees are facing difficulties with regard to facilities for education, medical care and drinking water. *Kachcha* wells are the main source of drinking water to them. As mentioned earlier the pattern of village settlements in the area is of houses built at a distance from each other. Generally tribals and Scheduled Castes stay in their own *tola* away from the main *abadi* settlement. In the circumstances even when one or two wells are constructed by the government or block agency these really do not serve the purpose of all inhabitants. Facilities for education and medical care are wanting and therefore, ayurvedic, homoeopathic doctors sometimes not even licenced are found commonly in the area. A few cases of the demand of Rihand displaced families are indicative of the needs of the area :

(i) In village Musrabehra, Panika locality has no school and their children have to go to school about two kms. away across a *nala* which is difficult to cross during rains. Hence there is a demand for a primary school in the locality.

(ii) In a locality near Babhni, Kols said that they get drinking water from a nearby *nala*, hence arrangement for drinking water should be made.

(iii) At Sukkhan, inhabited by Baigas, an old well has dried up and now people face a lot of problems in procuring drinking water. These families demand one hand pump for their habitation.

Overall, the problems are :

(a) Shifting from Rihand was unplanned and in a sense inhuman as people had to run along with their belongings and cattle.

(b) Transportation was inadequate and people had to carry their luggage for long distances.

(c) Land allottees were not given *patta*.

(d) Now survey agency is a source of tension for the tribals and the poor. Their land is being snatched away.

(e) There has been no follow-up of whatever rehabilitation policy was adopted for Rihand

oustees, specially in case of those settled away from the periphery of lake.

(f) Trafficking in women has increased on account of the influx of contractors and outsiders.

(b) Singrauli

The NTPC Singrauli has five main rehabilitation colonies/villages. Out of them the Chilkadand colony is a thickly pupulated one. Colonywise description is as follows :

Chilkadand

In this colony mainly displaced families of NTPC and NCL have been settled. It is said that a vast forest area was cleared and upland was levelled in order to form a rehabilitation colony. Plots of the size of 50′ □ 30′ were demarcated and plans for roads, lanes, etc. were laid. In 1977 the displaced families of NTPC were allotted house plots and people started settling down here and some who did not get plot settled on their own on the outskirts of the colony near a hillock.

It is now a very big settlement with population estimated to be more than 5000. It has two hamlets, Ranibari and Nimiyadand. A total number of nineteen communities live in the colony (Table 5.1).

The displaced families have mostly come from villages Gaharwar, Maanpur, Mushwasi, Hinoti, Kota, Ranibari, Dipa Pahri, Gharsadi, Batwa-Bhatwari, Raja Paraswar and Chaube Paraswar.

The colony is situated very close to the Shaktinagar railway station but there is no proper approach road to it. One has to cross the railway line and during rainy season one has to negotiate rain water which fills up the depressions near the railway line to reach the village. A market of the same name is situated on the right hand side of the main road connecting Anpara and Shaktinagar. Shops in the market are haphazard and mostly outsiders from Mirzapur, Varanasi and Haryana are the owners of the cloth, general merchandise and grocery shops, tea stalls, etc. In between the colony and the

TABLE 5.1 : **Community-wise Families in Chilkadand**

Sl. No.	Community	Number of Families (estimated)
1.	Kol	30
2.	Baiga	12
3.	Panika	2
4.	Kharwar	7
5.	Chamar	150
6.	Dhobi	6
7.	Koiri	40
8.	Kumhar	8
9.	Teli	70
10.	Kahar	20
11.	Kewat	18
12.	Nai	6
13.	Gosai (Giri)	7
14.	Brahmin	30
15.	Thakur	15
16.	Agrarshi	16
17.	Baniya	12
18.	Kayastha	12
19.	Muslims	8
	Total	449

market runs, the railway line where shunting of coal wagons and goods trains is done almost throughout the day. At times this endangers the life of the inhabitants of the colony, specially children, and livestock. There has been demand from the colony people for an over-bridge on the railway track but so far it has not been built.

The Pradhan of Chilkadand informed that displacement of the people has changed their economic life as a majority of the population was earning their livelihood by agriculture and allied activities but now almost all of them have become landless and depend on service or labour on daily wage basis. Some families pick up coal from the railway track and sell it though this cannot be called a regular and honest source of earning. Regarding facilities in the colony, the project has provided one *pucca panchayat ghar*, one junior high school and one homoeopathic dispensary (all having absestos sheet roofing) and roads. More than one hundred India Mark II hand pumps have also been installed, but the water is unhygienic. Some families have dug their own wells. Electric poles have been provided in the colony but no electric connections have been provided except in the school and the house of the Pradhan. Allotments of shops in the business centres of the project has been given only to outsiders so far.

Those families who got employment in the project can be said to be satisfied. But a majority of PAPs could not get employment and they have to work as daily wage labourers. The people are purchasing food-grains from open market at high rates and the facility of a ration-shop (public distribution system) is not available. They have not been given ration cards. The inhabitants of Chilkadand and Kharia are facing a regular threat from the blasting of coal fields which have caused cracks in their houses. Another problem was connected with milch cattle kept by the residents. This is a paying occupation and quite a few people have started keeping buffaloes and cows for the purpose. But some lower officials of the project have started exploiting such people by impounding their cattle and releasing them only on payment of heavy fines.

NTPC had promised that they would provide regular jobs to all young persons from the displaced families. Further, they had assured that even middle aged persons would be absorbed as watchmen and for similar other jobs. They had also held out that the colony would have all the amenities like roads, electric light, school, medical facilities, community centres, etc. The actual position is that only a few persons have been provided regular employment. As regards shop and *gumti* (kiosk), only two persons from amongst the oustees have been given *gumtis*. The colony has almost no roads which results in water logging and great difficulty for the residents. When visited the colony was found to be having no metalled roads and brick *kharanja* (paving) only for some distance. The rest of roads were *kachcha*. The Chilkadand colony is situated across the railway line near the Shaktinagar Station and the line goes on southward to Singrauli. NTPC, in spite of repeated representations has failed to construct a proper road from the main Shaktinagar-Singrauli road with a railway crossing. NTPC officers do not entertain any complaint in the matter. Some of the residents have started disposing of their milch cattle thereby losing the good source of income due to the harassment from the NTPC officials and death of cattle on the railway track.

Rani Bari

Rani Bari is a hamlet of Chilkadand village with a population of about 500, half of which belong to the Scheduled Castes, thirty-five per cent Backward castes, ten per cent higher castes and five per cent tribals. In this settlement, families from villages Mashwasi, Shahpur, Ranibari (old), Kota, Barwa-Bhatwari, Chaube Paraswar, Hinauni, Ghargaon fort, Manpur, etc. have been relocated by giving house-sites. Almost all the families numbering about one hundred have faced two times displacement, the first being in 1960 due to the Rihand dam and the second by NTPC in 1977. This colony too has not been provided with proper roads and approach to the place during rains is quite difficult. One has to cross the railway line and at times to creep below the rail wagons to reach the colony and as such it involves risk to human beings as well as cattle. NTPC has installed five hand pumps for drinking water but during our survey three of them were found to be out of order and the water was also not good. Electricity has not been provided so far though electric poles were erected last year. Only the junior high school at Chilkadand is available for the education of children, hence some children take education from two private teachers by paying Rs. 20 each per month. Similarly one homoeopathic dispensary at Chilkadand serves this area also and thereby people feel neglected for health care. There is no facility for the cremation of the dead.

Nimiyadand

This rehabilitation colony is also a hamlet of village Chilkadand with a population of about 1000, the Scheduled Castes, Backward Castes, Other Castes and the tribals being roughly in the same proportion as in Rani Bari. The main Scheduled Castes are the Chamar and Dhobi. Kol and Panika constitute the tribal group. Backward castes include Teli, Kushwaha (Kunbi), Kahar, Nai and Gosain and in the general category are Brahmins, Biyars and Muslims. The displaced families from villages like Manpur, Shahpur, Gursadia, Hinauni, Gahargaon (fort), Chilkadand, Diapahri, Barwa-Bhatwari, Nimiagarai, etc. have been rehabilitated in this colony. These families faced two displacements, first in 1960 by the Rihand dam and the second in 1977 by NTPC. The colony is not connected with any road or link road and the lanes in the colony are mostly *kachcha* and drainage is also very poor, causing insanitation. NTPC had provided eight hand pumps in the colony but most of them remain out of order and people face acute shortage of drinking water. It has not been provided with electricity though electric poles are there. The school at Chilkadand is expected to serve the children of this colony as well, Similarly homoeopathic dispensary at Chilkadand serves this colony also which is inadequate and no community centre has been provided here. As far as the employment opportunities are concerned hardly five per cent could get jobs out of which some are employed by NTPC and others by contractors. The Scheduled Castes and tribals were sore that even those whose land was acquired have not been provided with jobs. The oustees were not satisfied with the compensation amount and many of them are yet to get compensation money for wells, houses, trees and 'Varg-4' forest land which they had been cultivating.

The colony has no separate place for cremation of dead. People were not satisfied with rehabilitative measures because roads, lanes, bylanes and drainage have not been provided. Another general problem which came to notice relates to blasting in Kharia coal fields causing damage to their existing houses and other assets. The two colonies, viz. Rani Bari and Nimyadand being hamlets of the main Chilkadand colony have been ignored for facilities like education, medical care, community centres, roads, etc. even when their population is substantial through relocation of families from several villages.

Raja Paraswar Colony

The colony in Raja Paraswar was established in the year 1981 by the NTPC. A total of 259 plots were given to the oustees in this colony. However, roads were constructed only in 1991 and the electric poles were erected in July 1992. The original village was Raja Paraswar now submerged in the Rihand dam. The second displacement of these people came in the year 1981 due to the NTPC project and they were settled in New Raja Paraswar. Now they are in the process of a third displacement due to the construction of a railway line by the UPSEB for its Anpara project. Most of the houses which are going to be acquired by the UPSEB belong to the Scheduled Castes. There is no medical facility available in the colony.

Rakhi-Bandhi

It is situated near Kharia where a group of Baigas numbering about twenty households, have taken shelter leading a semi-nomadic life. These people said that after displacement from Rihand they moved to this area and erected their huts and used to earn their livelihood by labour. But in 1987 the Railway Board ousted them and they had no alternative but to settle across the railway line unathorisedly on an uneven land, because they were not given any type of facility/plot in the shape of compensation. Before the first displacement, these families were living in village Mehri now under Rihand reservoir and they emphasised that they did not get any assistance either from the Railway Board or from any other source at the time of displacement by the Rihand Dam. They chose this area for resettlement in the lure that they would get some type of work, being in the vicinity of factory area. This group of Baiga families has not till date received any attention from any project or government authorities. The place where they are living at present is not worth-habitation and no facility of any kind is available to them.

Some important issues voiced in the discussions with the people and by the Pradhan, were as follows :

(i) Many persons have completed 240 days on muster-roll work in the NTPC project but they have not been appointed on regular basis which is against the rules. Similarly, a large number of PAPs were called for interview from time to time through employment exchange, Robertsganj but none has so far been appointed.

(ii) Default in payment of *pratikar* (tax due to the Gram Sabha) on the land belonging to Gram Sabha Kota which has been occupied by NTPC. According to the Pradhan the tax arrears are a substantial amount. In addition

there is the case of the Varg-4 forest land which too has been taken over by NTPC.

(iii) Some *gram sabha* land which has been occupied by the NTPC should have been used for college, hospital buildings, etc. as per the assurance of the then Union Power Minister. But that has not been done so far.

(iv) Subedar Prasad Singh, M.P. wrote repeatedly to the Railway Minister for the construction of a foot overbridge at Shaktinagar station which was sanctioned in 1989 and provision of a children's park in the rehabilitation colony Chilkadand. However, nothing has been done by the Railway Board so far.

(v) A list of fifty-two persons from Kota, nine from Rani Bari and 131 from Chilkadand who are eligible and qualified for getting jobs because their lands had been acquired was furnished to the NTPC at their request but nothing has been done.

(vi) A case was initiated in the year 1986 for providing individual electric connections to a number of persons living in the colonies. Many of them had completed the formalities. However, till May 1993, no connections had materialised.

(vii) Some outsiders have been cheating the simple tribals by assuring them that they would obtain compensation and jobs for them.

(viii) The NTPC had asked the Pradhan to sent them a list of persons to be helped for getting work with contractors in a prescribed proforma. The Pradhan has complied, sending a list of 240 persons from Kota, Rainbair, Chilkadand, Kharia and Paraswar Raja colonies in May 1989. It has received no attention thereafter.

(ix) The payment of compensation to most of the

families ousted by the NTPC has remained pending. A camp of the Special Land Acquisition Officer (S.L.O.) Pipri at Shaktinagar is needed for making final and full payment of compensation to these families.

(x) Most of the displaced families said that in getting compensation from S.L.O. Office Varanasi at least ten per cent amount had to be given as bribe to the lower officials. Further more, the poor and simple tribals and Scheduled Caste persons get loans from the block authorities only after giving bribes to gram sevaks (VDO).

(xi) It came out that in the beginning of the project (1977-78) a sizeable number of displaced persons got employment on muster roll basis but they were not absorbed in regular jobs.

Besides the above common issues there were a number of individual cases which mirrored the difficulties faced by the oustees :

(i) A Kahar was allotted a plot of 50′ × 30′ at Chilkadand by the project. He could not build the house over it because of financial problems and it was grabbed by the Pradhan who constructed a house over it. He had moved this matter in the court but no help from any quarter came to him.

(ii) A widow of Kumhar caste said that her husband got a job in the NTPC after much efforts in 1986 and he got a staff quarter also. In 1987 he died leaving a daughter. The widow had not been given any house-plot and she is being constantly pressurised by the NTPC to vacate the quarter without being provided a house-plot.

(*iii*) A Teli (disabled, whose right hand is paralysed) begged for a plot and livelihood.

(*iv*) A Dhobi is running a grocery shop with a loan of Rs. 10,000 from the Block. But the V.D.O. took Rs. 2,000 as bribe, thus affecting his business.

(*v*) Another Dhobi stated that though his appointment was made in 1977 he was not allowed to join duties. He made all possible efforts for getting the job but ultimately ended up doing manual labour on daily wages.

(*vi*) A Chamar who worked for two years in NTPC on muster-roll and for six months as gardener was not provided with regular employment or a house plot.

(*vii*) A Panika was assured *patta* of house plot by Tahsil Lekhpal and his wife got a vasectomy done on herself in Dudhi as desired by the official but neither the *patta* of house plot nor pending compensation was given to him.

(c) Anpara

The rehabilitation colony, Dibulganj, is the largest one for Anpara oustees. Plots (60′ × 40′) have been provided here after cutting and levelling of forests and rocky area. Even to this day the colony has not been provided with roads, lanes, drains and electricity which account for insanitary conditions in the colony. Even *nullahs* and big pits have not been levelled causing stagnation of water. Its population is about 3,000. The displaced families are mostly from Kuldumri, Anpara, Audi, Kakri and Parasi. Drinking water facilities are inadequate because cutting of rocks is difficult and no blast wells have been constructed. The project authorities have provided a school, a dispensary and a *panchayat ghar*.

Regarding facilities available in the rehabilitation colonies, the project claimed that the colonies had roads (*kachcha* and *pucca*), drains, drinking water (through open wells, hand pumps and pipe lines), play-grounds, schools, medical facilities and electricity facilities. Eighty-four respondents out of 89, felt satisfied about educational facilities and sixty-five said that a dispensary (homoeopathic/ayurvedic) was available. However, a sizeable number, twenty-three (25.08%) reported that drinking water facilities were not adequate. Other amenities like roads, drainage and electric light were stated to be absent in the colonies by all the respondents.

Almost all the families opined that displacement had affected their social, religious and economic life. Further, they all said that they had not been provided with any better alternative source of livelihood except work with the contractors and in the new set-up their religious ceremonies, role of the traditional tribal priests and age old economy based on agriculture has been adversely affected. The coal mines project of Kakri, adjacent to Anapara Project, presently provides work to a few Anapara oustees.

(d) Northern Coal Fields Limited (NCL)

The NCL is located in a vast area stretching about 30-35 kms. from Anpara to Shaktinagar, and includes Bina, Kakri and Khadia coalfields. The PAPs in this belt include oustees by NCL, NTPC as well as railways, roads and high tension electric lines. These oustees have been settled or have settled on their own in villages/colonies like Ambedkar Nagar (old Balia-nala), Khadia, Jawaharnagar, Bansi, Parasi.

Ambedkarnagar

This rehabilitation colony has been established by the NCL and the name was given in 1982. Its population consists of about sixty per cent Scheduled Castes, thirty per cent Backward Castes and nine per cent tribals. The Scheduled Castes are represented by the Chamar; the

Backward Castes by Teli, Nai, Lohar, Koiri and the tribals by the Kharwar and Gond. The families here were earlier living in Babu Paraswar, Raja Paraswar, Kharia and Chilkadand villages. They faced the first displacement in 1960 on account of Rihand Dam and settled in Meritola of Kharia village, and subsequently from 1981 the NCL had been trying to shift them to the present place i.e. Balia-nala (Ambedkar Nagar). Originally the NCL authorities wanted to shift the families to Chanduwar colony in Bina but people opposed this move tooth and nail. It was learnt that the NCL authorities in order to remove them adopted a stern attitude and those who were working on muster roll basis were threatened with terminations. Only then some of them agreed to take compensation and shift to the new place. One such letter of threat was seen by us. However, the oustees were demanding house plots, compensation and employment before actually shifting. This process of confrontation continued for about a decade, say from 1981 to 1991. Ultimately the NCL authorities lured some workers to agree by giving them plots and launched a drive to force the PAPs to vacate the area by bull-dozing their houses in June 1992. This event caused a lot of terror in the area and the sufferers claimed, on an average, to have lost property worth Rs. 20,000 and whatever was left of their belongings was transported to Balia-nala in NCL dumpers in a callous manner. After this people had to move to the present place to retain whatever belongings were left. Even after this inhuman and cruel act some families were directed to move to Chanduwar colony, but even to this day people are waiting to get a plot at Balia-nala and are not at all prepared to go to Chanduwar. They have been living even in temporary sheds of tarpauline by the side of a hillock or footpath.

The oustees have not been given any type of employment except those who were already working on muster roll basis. So far about one hundred plots for housing have been given and the remaining families are living in trying conditions. Thus the colony gives a look of extended slum area rather than planned rehabilitation. Insanitary conditions dominate the scene. So far the colony has been provided only with *kuchcha* roads which become difficult to negotiate during rainy season and the area where the tribals are living is the worst part of the colony. A wooden plank on Balia-nala serves as a temporary bridge linking the *'adivasi basti'*. Wells for drinking water are still under construction and four hand-pumps have been installed out of which one is out of order. Electric poles have been erected on roads but the lights seldom work and no domestic connections are given. In some places drains have been taken up for constructions and facilities for education and medical care are absent. The people were extremely dissatisfied about not getting final payment of their compensation from the NCL and some have filed cases in law courts. Illegal impounding of cattle by some NTPC guards is usual and heavy blasting in coalfields is a continuous process around them. It causes constant fear, cracks in walls and loss of goats and other cattle. No place has been earmarked for disposal of dead.

Kharia

The rehabilitation colony of Kharia is located on both sides of the main road connecting Shaktinagar and Anpara. It extends upto the railway line on one side and upto the banks of Rihand on the other. On the road side shops, stalls and temporary sheds have sprung up along with permanent structures of shops of cloth, general merchandise, paints, auto-parts, etc. Its history goes back to 1960-61, when displaced families from Rihand took refuge in this area and their rehabilitation took place in a haphazard manner. However, since the area was largely open and people were having agricultural lands the living conditions were not cramped and of a rural character. In 1977 after the acquisition of land by the NTPC a phase of second displacement started. A few families were ousted by the U.P. Public Works Department also for road construction. Some were ousted by the railways for laying the rail track and they shifted to the main Kharia village. Thus, this area witnessed uprooting of families by both the NTPC and the NCL and others. The NTPC acquired land for rehabilitation of oustees by giving some more plots. The original inhabitants of the village also constructed houses and shops for renting. A good number of migrants from Varanasi, Mirzapur and other places have also settled here as the business is good. Some 200 families were ousted from here in June 1992 and shifted to Ambedkar Nagar by the NCL.

The displaced families have come from several villages, viz. Barwa-Bhatwari, Paraswar-Raja, Paraswar Chaube, Khrauli, Murrak-Bansi, etc. Kharia is a big village which is made up of Kharia proper, habitation across the rail track, Kharia-Mor (turning), northern and southern Kharia. The population is made up of more than a thousand households. This population includes about 40 per cent outsiders who have settled here for business, contract and allied works. The PAPs accounted for about 700 families. But on account of some subsequent shiftings the present number has been reduced to about 250 households. Amongst the rehabilitated, the caste-wise break-up is about sixty per cent Backward Caste represented by the Teli, Kumhar, Nai, Kunbi, Ahir and Kewat; twenty per cent Scheduled Castes—Chamar and Dhobi; ten per cent tribals, mostly Panika; and others mainly Bania and Brahmin. Under the rehabilitation scheme plots of the size of 50′ × 30′ have been given to most of the families, but some families have not got it and they are living in temporary sheds, huts and/or on rent. About five per cent of the displaced families have been provided employment with the projects and the remaining eke out their living by other means, overwhelmingly labour. The Kharia rehabilitation colony has not been provided with drinking water, drains, lanes and other facilities by the project. People have their own wells and hand pumps for drinking water. One primary school functions in the colony, but there is no dispensary. The problems of blasting as well as forcible impounding of cattle exist here as well. No separate place is earmarked for the disposal of the dead. Kharia as a composite village gives an impressive look from the road with *pucca* shops and houses but the interior portion, particularly the rehabilitation colony, presents an unhygienic and filthy atmosphere devoid of lanes, drains and slum-like growth of houses on the plots. On the whole, the tribals and the Scheduled Castes have little share in the business and other activities going on here.

Chanduwar

This colony has come up on the upper portion of the old village Chanduwar which was submerged in the Rihand reservoir, where the displaced families of Rihand had taken shelter in 1960-61. The NCL acquired the land of this village in 1979-80. NCL has provided employment to some high caste persons but others 'were not considered' and so is the case with compensation. The colony has not been provided with basic amenities like drinking water, light, school, dispensary, roads, etc. These difficulties and the rocky and high location of the plots dissuaded the PAPs from shifting to this colony, particularly from Ambedkar Nagar. Blasting by Bina Coald-field is a continuous threat to the life and property of the residents of this area.

Jawahar Nagar

This colony is situated between Chanduwar and Gharsani. About 900 sites of 60′ × 40′ size have been plotted out in which about one hundred families from Hardhoa *basti* and fifty from Kharia were settled. The population is made up almost entirely of Chamar families and five Teli and two Marwari Bania households. About fifty families from Hardhua were provided employment by the NCL Bina Project on the basis of loss of their lands but the families from Khadia are still waiting for jobs. The colony has been provided with basic amenities of drinking water (wells and hand pumps), roads, drains and one primary school. Electric poles have been fixed and a dispensary too has been provided but it does not function. Shops have been built but not allotted so far. Blasting around here is also usual. Though the colony is better planned and provided with basic amenities, its one drawback of location across the main railway line near Shakti Nagar railway station with no level crossing is so overwhelming that life here is both difficult and risky. The approach is a depression below the railway line which gets water-logged throughout the rainy season.

Barwani (Jamsila)

This colony came up on the upper portion of the old village Barwani which submerged in the Rihand reservoir in 1960. Some families from Barwani, Gharsani, Barkhor and Gaharwar villages settled here after the submergence. In 1979-80 NCL Bina displaced some families but so far no plots have been made or allotted and people live very close to the old site in pitiable conditions. The population is made up of about one hundred Biyar; ten Brahmin; five Sunar; ten Nai; ten Teli and five Kewat households. The colony lacks facilities like drinking water, dispensary, lanes and drains and light. However, one primary school is there. Apart from all this, blastings and illegal impounding of cattle is the main problem of the residents.

Bansi

This is on the east of road leading to Shaktinagar. In the beginning families from village Gaharwar, Bahewa, Pipri,

Bina, Bansi, Pharidand, etc., affected by the Rihand Project, settled at this place in 1960. Later, in 1976 NCL Bina acquired the land and uprooted a large number of families. So far no resettlement of displaced families has been done as plots have not been laid out and PAPs are living on their own. However, compensation for land has been received by most of them. The pending cases generally relate to houses, wells, trees, etc. The population is made up of about one hundred Panika; fifteen Kharwar; fifteen Bania; five Thakur and one Nai families. Hardly ten per cent displaced families could get jobs in the NCL. The area has been provided with drinking water facilities and a primary school by the Gram Sabha. But lanes/roads, drains, dispensary, electricity and community centre/ *panchayat ghar* are lacking.

Rehta

This colony is situated about three kms. east of Kakri village. It has both old and new habitations. The old one is of settlers from Rihand submergence and the new area has been created by the Kakri Coalfields (NCL) where families displaced from Gharsani, Rehta, Khori, Kakri, Sirsi and a few other villages have been settled in 1979-80. Its population is made up of about 500 households out of which Chamar have 300 households, followed by Gonds (100), Kharwar (15), Brahmin (10) and Nai, Lohar and Teli (20). The displaced families have been given plots of 60′ × 40′ size over which they have constructed houses but some of them are yet to get plots. In the name of basic amenities, hand pumps and wells, though inadequate, one primary school and patches of roads and drains exist. Lighting, dispensary, *panchayat ghar* are all lacking. On the whole the colony presents a look of better layout with plots but insanitation and filth mar it.

Parasi

This village is spread out in a big area. A part of it has

been earmarked for rehabilitation, where plots of 60′ 40′ size have been made and allotted to displaced families but many families particularly Chamars and tribals whose lands were acquired by the Renusagar Power House (UPSEB) have not been given plots. The population here is over 5,000 of which nearly two-thirds are Backward Castes (Ahir, Lohar, Teli, Nai, etc.), three per cent tribals (Kharwar and Panika); twenty-five per cent Chamars and the rest Brahmin and Bania. The colony has been provided with electricity, roads, drinking water and a school. But since it is a part of the big village and there are still a large number of families without proper plots or houses, its overall look is that of an unplanned habitation.

Thus this chain of rehabilitation colonies for the PAPs presents a depressing look of being disorganised, slum-like "with barren, dirty and overcrowded environment. It soon became apparent that the actual concept of the rehabilitation colonies was flawed and characterised by a lack of technical know-how and inadequate resources, insufficient even for the modest objectives which had been set. The promises about schools, roads and dispensaries have rarely been kept . . . colonies have undergone a process of marginalisation from the very moment when they were designated to be taken out of the mainstream. The colonies were situated away from towns and centres of activity . . ." (EDF 1990).

The coalfield areas nearby are busy with loading and unloading of coal by trucks and whirlwind movements of overhead cable trolleys. The roads and houses thus become black with coal-dust and the environment remains polluted with it. This causes health hazards to the unprotected people. Constant movement of wagons and trains forces them to mostly crawl below them to go out of the colonies. Then the danger arising out of powerful blastings is constant and quite unnerving to the populace. It often causes damage to their property for which no redressal seems to be available.

The main problem of displacement is caused by vast areas of acquisition and like NTPC the NCL authorities too tend to acquire much more than required area under the Coal Bearing Areas Act, 1957. Some informants in Parasi area said that in the year 1978-79, the Officer incharge of CCL (old name) wanted to acquire a vast area of land by enforcing a master plan. A court case was fought jointly by the affected families and it was decided on February 4, 1994 in favour of the local people and thus the master plan could not be applied. But even this was not the end of the matter and some cases are still going on since 1985 under the Coal Bearing Areas Act. Representations from and discussions with the residents pin pointed some issues which are as follows :

(i) Joint Secretary, Department of Energy had held a meeting of the Planning and Coordination Committee on July 6, 1984 at Singrauli which was attended by senior officers from all the projects. He indicated in the maps certain areas out of the land acquired by the NCL for the Chilkadand rehabilitation colony. However, in contravention of this decision the NCL were constructing their staff quarters over this land.

(ii) The NCL has constructed a coal yard in the area adjoining the Chilkadand colony. This will mean that coal dust will be heavily polluting the atmosphere in the colony and people will become victims of serious diseases like T.B. and asthma.

(iii) The NCL notified an area of 540 acres under the Coal Bearing Areas Act and the Chilkadand rehabilitation colony falls under this area. This is unjustified as people who were rehabilitated by NTPC will be displaced once again. It is

also pointed out that even though NTPC's plant area adjoins this notified area, it has not been included in the notification.

(iv) The houses in the Medritola hamlet of Kharia and Chilkadand belonging to the tribals and Scheduled Castes were bulldozed by the NCL in June 1992. The people were told that a compensation of Rs. 10,000 and a plot to each house owner would be arranged in fifteen days. This has still not been done.

(v) There is a list of 357 persons who suffered damages due to blastings by the NCL Kharia on January 21, 1992. The list includes two persons whose houses were extensively damaged and one of them was injured as well, while in remaining cases the walls of the houses got cracked. However, no relief has been made available so far.

(vi) The Kharia project has been paying compensation of land at the rate of only Rs. 7700 per acre whereas, some land in the area had been sold to the NCL by NTPC Singrauli at the rate of Rs. 34714.20 per acre.

(vii) In a meeting at Pipri Guest House on January 5, 1988, the area's M.P. suggested that the compensation of Rs. 7700 per acre must be increased. This was not approved by the General Manager (G.M.), Kharia on the specious plea that compensation to ninety-five persons had already been disbursed on the old rate and an increase now would not be proper. But the fact is that the NCL, in their Amlori project, paid compensation at the rate Rs. 4600 per acre in 1982, and in 1988 enhanced the rate to Rs. 19714.20 per acre adjusting the amounts paid earlier.

(viii) G.M. Kharia called some persons of the

Chilkadand colony on March 3, 1987 and threatened them. Therefore a delegation of local people met the U.P. Home Minister at Lucknow. They were assured that no injustice would be done to them and the Home Department wrote a letter to the district administration on this point. The S.D.M. Robertsganj visited the area on March 9 and he too assured that after displacement they would be properly settled at Balia Nala. But the NCL, on its own, wants to settle the displaced families in village Gharsani and Chanduwar which is outside Kharia project, about 10 Kms away near the Bina project and does not suit the PAPs at all.

A meeting was held at the NCL on July 18, 1982 headquarters at Singrauli, in which representatives of the cultivators, officers of the CCL and the local M.P. were present, to finalise the rate of compensation for lands acquired under the Coal Bearing Area Act, 1957. According to an affidavit given by Ram Pyare Panika, in this meeting an agreement was arrived at on the following points :

(a) Full compensation on agreed terms must be paid immediately since the cost of land may increase later on.

(b) Land rate was fixed at Rs. 7700 per acre and it was also agreed to pay for land under *Varg* 4 (forest land).

(c) Officers of the CCL would distribute the compensation money.

(d) Compensation for houses, trees and other assets, like wells, *bandhis* would be given at the prevailing market rates.

(e) In the agreement, many points were not

recorded and it was also not considered necessary to record that the above rate would be applicable to those who will be paid compen-sation in that very year. The M.P. had opined that the compensation rates should be in accordance with market rate prevailing in the year of payment.

(*f*) All displaced families should be provided house plots of 60′ × 40′ size and the rehabilitation colonies should be provided with electricity, water, hospital, etc.

The above agreed terms obviously remained unfulfilled and had to be restressed in a meeting of the Rehabilitation Cell held on April 5, 1986 which was presided over by the M.P. It was attended by the officers of the Coal Projects, S.D.M. Dudhi, A.D.M. Mirzapur, other Revenue Officers and the Gram Pradhans of Parasi, Kharia, Rehta and other villages. Some other vital issues brought up in this forum were :

(*a*) Compensation rate should be raised on the analogy of other projects.

(*b*) The order that displaced families would not be provided jobs should be withdrawn.

(*c*) The displaced families must be rehabilitated within the project area.

It was also decided that the cultivators should always be informed by notice of the land to be acquired under Section 7 of the Coal Bearing Areas Act and this land should be taken by the projects only after paying the compensation.

But even after a lapse of seven years the terms of the agreement were not honoured and the PAPs were given a step motherly treatment. This is borne out by a report in the *Swatantra Bharat* dated January 26, 1989. It states that the NCL project had not provided employment to the displaced families and no electricity was provided in the colony at Rehta. Many displaced families were facing the problems of hunger and some unemployed youths of Rehta village had met the Senior General Manager of Kakri Project for getting some work in coal grading plant. But they were abused and shown the door whereas in this very plant the coal transport companies were regularly employing people from outside.

The foregoing account gives a clear idea about the problems and treatment meted out to the displaced families. The main problems can be summarised as below:

(i) Most of the families have not been provided with any source of earning or livelihood.

(ii) Colonies of rehabilitation do no present a look of planned layout and basic amenities are singularly lacking.

(iii) Outside labour is preferred over the local displaced persons.

(iv) Compensation for trees, houses, etc. has not been paid even after displacement and many families did not get plots for housing. Documents which came to our notice showed that the compensation for a house was assessed at Rs. 127 only in one case and usually the *mahuwa* (*Madhuea indica*) trees have been valued at Rs. 10 for compensation!

(v) Blastings by the coal fields are a constant threat to life and property of the families.

(vi) Forcible eviction and even bulldozing of houses are common in the area.

(vii) At present, for the labour jobs of the NCL an I.T.I. diploma is compulsory. Some young boys from the displaced families who had such diplomas were appointed as apprentice for one year, but they were not absorbed in

regular jobs.

(viii) Some NCL officials demanded Rs. 20-25 thousand for giving employment as labour.

(ix) There was a constant fear of being displaced in the minds of all residents of the area, as more coal bearing tracts are likely to be identified.

(x) Infrastructure, like rail-line for transporting coal, high-tension electric lines and roads are still under construction causing further displacements.

(xi) The tribals and Scheduled Castes who were dependent on agriculture and forests are particularly unable to adjust to the changed economic life and no specific efforts to rehabilitate them came to notice.

(xii) Even the landless oustees claim that they had 'become *Bhumihin*', meaning thereby that their livelihood as agricultural labourer, share-cropper, etc. had been lost.

(e) Bijpur

The Project created two rehabilitation colonies in Bijpur known as Punarvas Colony 1 and 2. Plots of size 60′ × 40′ were demarcated after levelling rocky and hilly areas and cutting of forest. This land was also acquired from the local people for rehabilitation purpose. In the colony, some metalled roads and short distance *kharanja* (brick paved) roads have been laid. A primary school and a *panchayat-ghar*, has been constructed by the project. Some houses or plots have not been linked with the roads so far. The area of the colony is undulating and during rainy season low lying areas get water logged. Twenty hand pumps and six wells were provided by the project and a plan of piped water supply is afoot. However, the residents of colony informed that almost all hand pumps had gone out of order and four wells too had gone dry, thereby causing much difficulty in getting drinking water. An overhead tank on the top of hillock with a pipeline has been laid, but it has not yet become functional because of technical flaws and people call it 'a drama' because the overhead tank is said to be defective. A private high school is also being run in a rented building by an out-sider from Robertsganj. So far the colony has not been provided with electric connections, though the project gave connection to the police station, very near the colony. On this issue people are very much annoyed. One of the informants said that the project authorities said that domestic connections were in the purview of UPSEB and the NTPC were concerned with production of energy only.

Medical and entertainment facilities have not been provided. People go to the private doctors in the market or a centre run by the Banwasi Seva Ashram at Chetwa, a nearby village. In the beginning treatment and medicines were provided to the displaced families by the project hospital. Now this has been discontinued and charges for medicines are now taken. An aged carpenter (*Barhai*) told us that in 1988-89 a training programme of carpentry for about two years was run by the project in the primary school building. He had worked as trainer and eighteen trainees completed their training. Now the centre has been closed and all material and equipments have been removed. He further informed that once Vasant Sathe, the Union Energy Minister, had visited the colony and listened to their problems. He sounded very considerate and sympathetic towards the difficulties, particularly regarding facilities in the colony and people's livelihood. He had asked the General Manager of the project to ensure piped water supply to every house and get *pucca* platforms constructed outside the houses in the colony, similar to that of project quarters. Further, the unemployed youth should be given monthly allowance till they were absorbed in regular work. But practically nothing has been done.

If a comparison of this colony is made with those of Shakti Nagar, Anpara, Bina and Bansi, this colony's layout is better, with no overcrowding. Two displaced families, one Teli and another Brahmin, have recently been allotted places for setting up flour mills (*atta chakki*) and *pan* shop (betal-cigarette) in the shopping centre of the project. But, excepting this, all types of work under contract, shops, kiosks, etc. have been allotted to outsiders.

Visthapit Morcha, an organisation formed in this colony has been demanding the much needed facilities for the colony and jobs in the NTPC. Incharge of Banwasi Sewa Ashram at Chaetwa said that till July, 1992 only 128 persons had been provided employment as class IV employees by the project. However, those displaced families whose one acre or more land had been taken were assured jobs—one person per family in other works like contract work, allotment of shops, labour preference etc.—but the assurances have not been adhered to. In an affidavit filed by the NTPC in 1984, only nine local people were stated to have been employed by them. However things improved afterwards due to the efforts of non-government organisations like the Banvasi Sewa Ashram and Visthapit Morcha and the Supreme Court's judgement in a case filed by the Ashram.

The Bijpur area has witnessed a second chain of displacements with the setting up of NTPC's Super Thermal Power Project in 1982, the first being in 60s on account of Rihand. The problems of displacement and rehabilitation are as follows :

(*i*) Affected families' land, house, etc. were taken without the launching of a proper resettlement plan for the oustees.

(*ii*) Compensation was not paid within the stipulated period and even after a lapse of ten years, some people have not been paid full amount for their houses and trees and forest land under their cultivation recorded as *'Varg-4'* by the revenue department.

(iii) Plots were made after much delay, resulting in a lot of inconvenience to the displaced families.

(iv) Transportation of household goods, tiles, roofing material, etc. was done in a haphazard way causing huge losses to the displaced families and some families were not helped in the shifting.

(v) Ouster from their original homes was expedited by extensive bulldozing of the PAPs houses but no plots were ready for them by that time to enable them to settle down.

(vi) Compensation money could not be utilised for house-construction as plots were allotted seven or eight years after displacement in some cases. Even now *pattas* have not been given to the plot allottees. All this retarded the progress in house building activity in the rehabilitation colony.

(vii) In giving compensation, the tribals, particularly who were illiterate and ignorant, were cheated by middle men and others.

(viii) No rehabilitation programme for the landless and artisan families has been thought of by the NTPC so far.

(ix) The training programme in carpentry also did not help the trainees in getting jobs or self employment and it was given up too soon.

(x) Loss of agricultural lands virtually left the PAPs without any assured source of livelihood all of a sudden. Earlier, agricultural work used to absorb all family members, young and old, in different pursuits. Now not more than one person per family is in job and others have no source of earning except to look for casual labour work. Jobs too have been provided to

only a few.

(xi) Now, people are buying foodstuff, etc. from shops on credit because most of them have spent the compensation money already.

(xii) A few who ventured into small business of grains, grocery, suffered losses due to the influx of people from outside in this trade who had better resources and business sense.

(xiii) Displaced families have not been given their due in the allotment of shops, contracts, etc. and outsiders were preferred. In the Bijpur bazar of the project campus, 307 plots for shop were made out. Grave irregularities have been committed in the allotment of these shops (*Ghati Ka Dard* 1988).

(xiv) The PAPs are facing difficulties in getting fuelwood because the forest department harasses those collecting dead wood.

(xv) Some time back Kalpnath Rai, the then Union Energy Minister had visited the Bijpur PAPs colony. He had assured them of adequate drinking water supply and electricity within a short period. But the promise remains unfulfilled.

(xvi) A *dharna* started at the gates of the Bijapur project by the PAPs to highlight the indifference and unhelpful attitude of the project authorities could not bring about any sympathetic response from them. The PAPs have been fighting for the last ten years and have a fourteen-point charter of demands. The project has so far totally ignored even the genuine grievances, viz. electric connection, drinking water facilities, an intermediate college in the area, ponds/ tanks for cattle, jobs, training and other opportu-nities for alternative employment, shops in the project complex, house plots for

persons left out, free treatment in the project hospital, payment of balance compensation and banning construction of houses by unauthorised persons in the colony.

In may be mentioned again that the authorities of this project refused to provide for this study any data whatsoever regarding the rehabilitation measures taken by them and the plans, if any, prepared in that connection. Furthermore, we were surprised over the attitude of the second top-most executive of the project when he 'claimed' in a personal discussion that, the setting up of the project in this area had 'civilized the inhabitants'. When we asked him to elucidate how this was happening, he said that these people had never even seen a motor truck or electric light before the project came on the scene.

(f) Kanhar

Actual displacement has not taken place as yet in this project area. The project authorities have not provided any house sites (plots) or colonies for the displaced families, as found in other clusters. Comparatively, complaints about bribe, etc. are few and people are in an advantageous situation since they still cultivate the acquired land and labour work is easily available on the earthen dam and its canals. Thus, the impact of Kanhar project is not evident so far except people's complaint that the area is still devoid of irrigation facilities, besides some irregularities in the payment of compensation and grouse against disturbance to cultivators and other work by the survey teams of the project.

The project has not provided basic amenities to those families whose lands have been acquired. Schools, hospitals, roads, electricity, etc. that exist here were provided by the departments concerned. Only five of the surveyed families had domestic electric connections.

Pucca roads and link roads are few and mostly *kachcha* roads are available. People apprehend that after filling up of the dam, their style of life may change as the facility of cultivation will go, and demand that one member of each family should be provided regular employment by the project and the rate of land compensation must be equal to what has been given in Bijpur area, viz., Rs. 10,000 per acre. Our inquiries with the project authorities revealed that there has been little planning or preparation for proper and stable resettlement of the people who would be displaced when the dam is filled up with water.

The factors responsible for such dismal conditions in the rehabilitation colonies were identified as indifference of the project authorities even to the minimal needs of the rehabilitated persons, their inaccessibility for any redressal of grievances, a patent lack of coordination among the government departments like the railways, public works, rural engineering, etc. and the project authorities and the lack of will on the part of the latter to press the govern-ment agencies for effectively playing their role. Further, another significant part of the story was that the rehabilitation colonies today present some kind of a "grey area" in so far as the jurisdiction, control and responsibility of the various agencies concerned go. The project authorities are supposed to invest in the infrastructural work in a colony but what will be the position when the rehabilitated people relate to more than one project or with regard to the proper maintenance of the facilities. Similarly in certain villages the PAP families came and settled subsequently. So they are not treated as the inhabitants of the village in question. The panchayat jurisdiction has also not been extended to these extended 'abadi' areas and in any case the panchayats do not have resources to create amenities in the *tolas* inhabitated by the PAPs. In spite of the demand made by the panchayats neither the projects nor the government care to provide even a part of the substantial funds required for the purpose. Even though decades have passed the readjustment in the boundaries of the panchayats has not been done on the basis of the ground situation. The entire picture has continued to be in a position of flux and confusion. The settlers themselves are, therefore, in a state of insecurity and uncertainty whether they should continue to live there or move away to some other places where they can find a better environment.

6

VOICES OF THE OUSTEES

THE project-wise details of the extent of displacement, rehabilitation measures, compensation and some socio-economic indices of the oustees' existing state were presented in the last chapter. It was based on an extensive family-wise survey. In this chapter, a kaleidoscopic picture of the empirical situation is analysed. The reality has been projected through focused autobiographies or we may call them cases. These cases reflect the perception of the people—one of the chief aims of the anthropologist is to understand the emic view—with regard to the whole gamut of circumstances they have passed through. In fact evaluation of development projects through case studies provides valuable qualitative information to analyse the situation (Patnaik 1990). Many recent studies have convincingly used this technique with regard to both rural development (Roy and Srivastava, 1986) and tribal development (Chaudhury 1993). Though the cases come through micro-level investigations, they represent the macro-level reality effectively. Care has been taken to select the cases in an objective manner so that they represent the whole universe. In total 31 cases have been presented here and they are followed by a discussion on the situation.

Case 1

CK of village Raja Paraswar belongs to the Panika

community, one of the tribal groups of the area. Panikas are traditionally cloth weavers. CK is fifty years old and has four daughters and one son, out of whom three daughters are married. His original village was Khairi, now submerged in the Rihand reservoir, where he had seven acres of land. He along with his father used to cultivate it till 1961, when it got submerged.

CK left for village Kogwar, district Surguja, M.P., after being displaced. There he had some relatives. He remained there for a few years but could not settle down to any occupation, due to lack of resources. However, his father had in the meantime got a housing plot and some agricultural land (area not specified) in village Nemna, four km. from Raja Paraswar, where he had started cultivation. While CK was in Surguja district his father expired and a neighbour belonging to the Baiswar caste (an influential caste in the area) forcibly grabbed the land, knowing fully well that CK would not be in a position to get it back since he belonged to a weaker section. After his father's death, CK returned and settled in Raja Paraswar in the year 1970 where he thought he could get some work as a labourer due to its proximity to the NTPC project.

The land in Khairi was in the name of his father who had received a compensation of Rs. 1900. CK does not know how his father had spent this money at that time. After coming to Raja Paraswar CK has built a house. He claims that the NTPC has acquired the house, but he has been told to continue living in it, which is the case with many other persons. Neither any compensation has been paid to him, nor has he been given a housing plot. He is working as labourer with a NTPC contractor on 'supply basis' since 1984. He gets work for about 22 days in a month and the current wages are Rs. 38.60 per day. Out of this Rs. 100 are deducted towards "Local Samiti Expenditure". He bitterly says that in spite of two displacements, he has not got a permanent job either through the Rihand Dam or NPTC. In the process of seeking a job, some government servants (not identified) advised him that he should get 'family planning operation' done for his wife and they would then secure a job for him. The operation was got done but no job was given. His wife is also supplementing the family income by running a tea stall on the road side. According to CK this effort has not yielded much profit mainly because they have no money to invest in the stall and improve it.

Nostagically remembering the past, CK said that before Rihand displacement his family was quite well-off 'prosperous in every way'. "Now, we are facing difficulties in every way and earning a living is very difficult". Moreover in the old village they were weaving cloth for traditional needs of the community, in addition to agriculture, which has now been given up totally. Describing the changes in the social system he says that Khairi was quite a well-to-do village. It had about one hundred houses of Baiswar, twenty houses of Rajput, ten houses each of Brahmin, Teli and Chamar and five houses of Panika. The village had a village deity *Baiga Deeh Dham* which was worshipped with a lot of fan-fare. Now, with the populace getting dispersed, the deity is no more worshipped. Other festivals were also celebrated with gaity.

Among the Panika there was no dowry system and marriages could be arranged without any difficulty. Now the practice of *Tilak Dahej* has come about and it has made it difficult for people like him to settle the marriage of their daughters. The practice of taking services of Brahmin, Baiga, Nai and Dhobi was there in the old village and has been continuing.

The colony in Raja Paraswar has been provided with hand pumps only a year back and the same is the case with electric lamp-posts. There is a government primary school and also a ration shop. However, the supply of ration is irregular and inadequate. There is no medical facility available in the colony.

Case 2

CH of Raja Paraswar who is seventy years old has faced two displacements—first in 1961 for Rihand dam and second in 1980-81 for the NTPC. He is a Dharkar, a Scheduled Caste. All of his children (five sons and two daughters) are married. He is illiterate. Originally he hails from village Marrak Bansi, about twenty km away from Raja Paraswar, which got submerged in Rihand reservoir. In that village he owned about two acres of land for which he received Rs. 300 as compensation in 1960. After submergence he first moved to an area near the hills along with others from his village. He was displaced again in 1980-81 by the NTPC, for which he got a total compensation of Rs. 6,000 and a house plot of 50′ × 30′ at Raja Paraswar. He has no land now and he is subsisting totally on casual labour.

CH recalls that he was getting good crops from his two acres of land which was irrigated from river Rihand. In addition, he pursued his traditional craft of making baskets, *sup* (winowing fan), etc. from bamboo and also worked for catechu contractors in preparing catechu during the season. Some people were also collecting fuel-wood from the forests nearby and selling it. Now, there is no forest in the vicinity of Raja Paraswar and hence no additional income can be had. The traditional bamboo craft of Dharkars is also now finished. He bitterly says that now he has become a 'beggar and even alms are not forthcoming'. It is extremely difficult for the family to get two full meals. According to him the Dharkars as a group are the worst sufferers as they cannot make their voice heard. "Whenever they are able to approach some 'factory-wala' the latter blatantly asks them to take to begging". In the old village of Marrak Bansi, there were about a hundred families each of Teli and Dharkar, twenty houses of Chamar, five houses each of Ahir and Panika, two houses of Brahmin and three houses of Rajput. CH said that a large number of people from his village moved to Madhya Pradesh and even Bihar and settled down wherever they could get a place.

Describing the changes that have come about, he says that previously there were caste *panchayats* which were looking after the well-being of the various caste groups. This system has now disintegrated and as a result castes, particularly the Dharkars, have lost their base (and leadership). Religious life and festivals have been totally disturbed and generally given up. There is no worship of *Baiga Dih* any more. The Dharkar continue to celebrate the Hindu festivals as in the past but in a very low key. People are very poor now and loss of lands has deprived them of the means to practice the rituals and celebrate festivals. Another change is a marked deterioration in the level of people's health. Previously, people were healthy and ordinary diseases were taken care of by the Baiga healer and his herbs and roots. Now the incidence of various diseases is high. In the colony the facility of hand pumps and internal roads as well as electric lamp-posts has been provided during the last one year only though it was inhabited several years ago.

Case 3

RP, a seventy year old Baiga, has faced four displacements. At present he lives with this family consisting of eleven members. He was first displaced from his original village Bichchi due to the Rihand Dam in the year 1960. Since he got no rehabilitation facilities, he started moving from one place to another and in 1964 he came to Raja Paraswar. Near this village he along with a few other Baigas, made huts in a hamlet called Rakhi Bandhi. They were supporting themselves only through casual labour. In the year 1983-84 they had to leave these habitations suddenly because Rakhi Bandhi area (called 'S.Dam') was innundated with water one night. They moved into Raja

Paraswar village school. At the time of innundation a Baiga woman and her small child were drowned and this was reported to the authorities. Subsequently the Tehsildar of Dudhi inspected the area and gave Rs. 100 per family to the people and asked them to build their huts in another part of Rakhi Bandhi. RP says that they had heard that some compensation was sanctioned for the two lives lost by drowning but no money ever reached the affected family. According to him "it must have been eaten up by the government functionaries; this is the fate of the adivasis".

The next displacement of these people came in the year 1990 due to the construction of railway line. Buldozers were used to remove their huts and for this displacement they got no compensation or shown any alternative habitation sites. Since then they have been living in a plot near the old place which belongs to RS, a Brahmin (it was gathered that RS had allowed the Baiga to put their huts, which were small and make-shift type, on his land which too had been acquired by NTPC and therefore the Baiga were liable to be thrown out any day). RP said that the Baiga ware supporting themselves with whatever casual labour came their way. They had no place to live and no assurance of help regarding their livelihood.

In their original village also the Baiga were largely landless but they were able to support themselves by becoming *halwaha* (ploughmen) with the agriculturists and taking up casual agriculture work. Besides, there were good forests around the village and they were able to collect and sell minor forest produce, fuel-wood, etc. Some people also helped the forest contractors in preparing catechu. This was a seasonal work yieldling reasonable wages. In the original village they had only small houses and the compensation received from Rihand project for the houses ranged from Rs. 50 to Rs. 150 which was spent in putting up huts elsewhere.

At present the condition of RP's family as well as the

other Baiga families living in Rakhi Bandhi is of extreme deprivation. He said that they had hardly any clothes, beddings or other household goods and managed to get one meal a day with difficulty. Sometimes even that is difficult and 'we have to do *upvaas*' (fast). RP emphatically said that he and his people never received any facility either from the NTPC or government excepting the small amount from Rihand mentioned earlier. According to him they have no leader who can draw the attention of the government or porjects to their sad plight, 'we are living like animals', he said.

Speaking of changes from past to the present, RP said that previously they used to elect a *Mukhia* for their *Biradari-Tat*. The displacements have scattered his people here and there and spelt the end of *Biradari Panchayat*. They also find it difficult to get matches for their girls and boys. People have moved far and wide and the traditional organisation, communication and marriage network has been disrupted. Due to this difficulty even dowry system has started making its appearance in place of bride-price. In the marriage the Baiga call Pandit, Nai and Dhobi and they still follow this practice.

In the original village the Baiga were well off because they were priests of the village *Deehwar* (place of deity). They also practiced as faith healers and sold herbs and other medicines. The traditional tribal festivals like Karma was celebrated with enthusiasm and so were other festivals like Holi and Ram Navami, etc. Now due to their utter poverty and day to day search for *roji-roti* (a living) the festivals are hardly celebrated. With the disappearance of forests, the work of collecting herbs and roots and providing traditional services of healing to their regular clientele has also suffered, almost ended.

Case 4

Forty-five years old JP is a Biyar by caste. He is illiterate and lives in Gharsani hills. He has a family of six including his mother, wife and three children. In his original village of Gharsani (plains) he had one and half acre of land. At the time of its submergence under Rihand the compensation for this land was fixed at Rs. 90 which was paid to JP's father. After submergence they moved up the hill and cleared some land and settled there. Thereafter the Bina Project of CCL initiated mining work in the area and surveyed their land in the year 1975. JP described that the survey was *'manmani'* (high handed) and the compensation fixed for them was also *'manmani'* ranging from Rs. 150 to 300. He was paid Rs. 150. Some more compensation remained to be paid but in the meantime the Brahmins of the village started claiming as theirs the land on the hills reclaimed by the Biyar and other weaker sections. This matter has been pending in the court of S.D.M. Pipri since then. As a result they have been denied alternative plot or compensation or job by the NCL. They are still living in the same place feeling very insecure as they are likely to be displaced any time either by the Brahmins or the NCL.

According to JP, in the original village the Brahmins were the dominant caste with seventy families and the Biyar had sixty houses. There were one hundred forty houses of the Chamar, twenty houses of Sonar, four houses of Bania and one house each of Teli and Lohar. There were also ten houses of Nai. The village community disintegrated on submergence. Some people left for Madhya Pradesh (Sarguja District) and some others moved towards Babhani. Out of the remaining people some have built their houses on the hill-top. JP said that Biyars were largely vegetable growers and horticulturists. They were quite prosperous even with their small patches of land. Some subsidiary income was obtained from the forests, collecting minor forest products like *mahuwa, amla,* lac and fuel wood. People were quite satisfied with their lot then.

The present circumstances are extremely harsh. Even

though there has been a big price rise, there is no assurance of any source of income for the Biyar. People coming from outside are getting work here at the cost of the local people, who are starving. They are unable to get even regular labour work with the labour contractors. On top of it they have been burdened with the litigation initiated by Brahmins.

The only facility given by the NCL is a hand-pump in their present village. Another hand-pump has been installed by the gram sabha. There is no ration shop and they have not been provided ration cards. JP also complained about the lack of medical facilities and non-availability of their commonly used medicinal herbs, roots, etc. due to disappearance of forests. Biyar's social organisation has been disturbed with the breaking up of *Biradari Panchayat*. The *Mukhias* are not being regularly elected and the *panchyat* is not functioning properly any more. Among Biyars, dowry is now being given at the time of *Tilak*. However, the use of the services of Pandit, Baiga, Nai and Dhobi are continuing. Previous-ly the Baiga used to build village *Deeh* where worship used to take place regularly and the villagers pros-pered. Now these practices have largely disappeared.

Case 5

HC, aged forty, lives in Jawahar Nagar near Chilkadand. He has a family of ten, which includes his wife, six sons, one daughter-in-law and one grandson. HC's caste is Chamar traditional leather workers, besides being an important community engaged as agricultural labourer. In his original village Nawka, near Chilkadand, which has been submerged under Rihand reservoir, he had fifteen acres of land. After the sub-mergence of his village he was provided with two acres of land as a Rihand oustee in village Hardhoa and Rs. 1500 as compensation. He settled there.

The land in Hardhoa was acquired by the NCL in the

year 1984-85. He got compensation at the rate of Rs. 7,000 per acre, totalling Rs. 14,000 and another Rs. 8,000 for his house and other possessions. As a result of this second displacement he became totally landless. He had to move to the Harijan Basti of Jawahar Nagar near the old village of Chilkadand where the NCL provided him a plot measuring 60′ □ 40′. He has got a job in the NCL but finds it difficult to support his large family from that income. He commented that the NCL has no fixed rules relating the quantum of land lost by the oustee to the provision of a job. Hardly about 50 per cent of oustees have been given jobs.

Remembering his old village he said that there were 200 houses of Chamar and some houses of Brahmins and Gosain, etc. Some of the Chamar families moved some where towards Muirpur. The village was situated on both sides of the river Rihand. The river water provided irrigation facilities and, therefore, their agriculture was quite good. The yield was enough for their own consumption and there was surplus for sale. In addition the people had access to the forests and collected fire-wood and minor forest products like *mahua, anwala*, lac, etc. Some of which was sold.

The village *Birdari* of the Chamar was a well-knit unit headed by *Biradari Mukhia*. This system has now been disturbed. The village also had a *Baigadeeh* and temples. Previously in the marriage there were traditional musical instruments going with the *Barat* and there were Pandit and Baigas traditionally attached to the families in a village. All these customs have undergone changes. Commenting on the facilities available to the persons living in his colony, he said that the hand-pumps were there but these were seldom in a working condition. Lamp-posts had been erected but the colony was dark and the approach roads to the colony usually got flooded with water. The colony had a primary school and also a dispensary. However, the dispensary had no doctor and no stock of medicines. The NCL have also not provided any area for building a temple or for cremation/burial. Another problem was of getting ration and kerosene oil. There was no ration shop and people had no ration cards. Instead of kerosene oil they had to buy diesel oil and use it for lighting their house. The NCL does not even arrange the supply of coal for fuel in their oustee colonies.

Case 6

HZ belongs to the Chamar caste. He is illiterate and sixty years of age. He is now living in the Harijan Basti of Chanduwar rehabilitation village. His family consists of twelve members including two sons, their wives and children. His original village was Gharsani about six km. away which has been submerged in the Rihand reservoir. There his father had two acres of land for which he got a compensation of Rs. 400 in the year 1961. They shifted from their village and for this purpose no facilities were provided to them except cash compensation. They had to face a lot of difficulty in moving to Chanduwar.

The second displacement came in the year 1982-83 when the place where he was living in Chanduwar village was acquired by the CCL (now NCL). NCL gave a compensation of Rs. 1700 but no other facilities such as a plot or job were provided to him. He complained that, by and large, the Brahmins managed to get better compensation while the Scheduled Castes suffered. The Brahmins got compensation even for their *banjar* lands. In the case of Scheduled Castes and weaker sections it was said that the land they were occupying 'belonged to the government and therefore no compensation was admissible'. The survey and measurements were done some twelve years ago but Scheduled Castes have till now got nothing. The Brahmins have, however, been provided jobs as well as compensation since then.

Remembering about his old village, HZ said that the

village had a population of Brahmins, Chamars, Gadarias and Biyars. There were a few houses of Sonar, Rajput and Koiri as well. Many of these persons moved to Surguja or Babhani while some settled down at the farthest end of the Rihand reservoir. Gharsani village was on the bank of Rihand river and therefore the quality of their agriculture was good. Some of the Scheduled Caste persons were engaged as *halwaha* or obtained land on *batai* basis. The access to forests ensured fuel-wood and some minor forest produce which supplemented their food and income. HZ stated that the *Panchayat Tat* of the Chamar has lost its importance and has almost died out. The *Panchayat* used to keep control over the marriage customs and therefore no dowry was in vogue. Now dowry had become a regular custom creating difficulties for poorer people. The worship of village deities has also been given up.

In the present locality the only facility provided to them is a hand pump. No school, dispensary or ration shop exist. Getting regular work on daily wages is also difficult for most of the people.

Case 7

RS is a Brahmin and is literate. He lives in village Barwani. He has a family of six including three daughters and one son, all unmarried and young. He hails from Gharsani which was submerged in Rihand reservoir in 1960. His father owned ten acres of land in Gharsani for which they got cash compensation of Rs. 2000. Thy moved to Barwani because his father owned some land there as well.

In 1979-80 NCL Bina acquired an area around Barwani, but RS was not affected since he had only the house which was not acquired. Persons whose agricultural land was acquired have been given compensation. According to RS the NCL had initially fixed the compensation at a low rate. Later the people agitated and the compensation was raised to Rs. 7,000 per acre which too was not fair. He also stated that those persons who did not possess clear title of their land had also been paid compensation at the rate of Rs. 2000 per acre. However, jobs have been given only to persons who owned larger pieces of land. He estimated that not more than 30 per cent of the affected persons in his village have been given jobs. Persons who have got jobs are comparatively in a better position. Others are facing difficulties because there is no agriculture left with them and labour work with contractors is the only source of income.

Remembering the past, he said that the village depended almost entirely on agriculture. His father and he along with two other brothers were quite well-off on their agricultural land. However, his brothers got jobs, one in NCL and the other in HINDALCO through some sources, but he could not manage to get a job and therefore he is in a very 'insecure economic condition' with young children, at the age of about fifty years. They were growing rice, potatoes, chillies, etc. on their lands and had enough surplus for sale. Besides, the forest provided fuel-wood and timber for housing as well as minor forest products like *amla, mahuwa,* lac, etc. In their original village people generally suffered from ordinary diseases which could be cured either by a *Vaid* or sorcery done by the Baiga. However, he felt that now the people were becoming prone to more serious diseases caused by pollution in the area. These complicated diseases are curable only by modern medicine but the common people are unable to afford such treatment. Further, the persons belonging to Biyar caste used to take good care of diseases of the cattle. With the dispersal of village population as a community, to different places, this service too is no more easily available. The newly set up rehabilitation colonies have no facility for the treatment of cattle.

Case 8

PR belongs to the Biyar caste. He is illiterate and fifty

years old. He has a large family of twenty two persons including his parents, four married sons and their children. He is living in Barwani near the NCL colony for oustees. His original village was Gharsani which was submerged in the Rihand reservoir. There he had two acres of land and the compensation that he got for it was Rs. 400. It was spent by his father only in shifting and settling down in Barwani in the year 1961. According to him, the family did not get any other rehabilitation help from the Rihand authorities.

At Barwani, they gradually acquired nearly ten acres of land during the two decades following the first displacement. Subsequently in 1980-81 his entire land was acquired by the NCL for coalfields and the compensation fixed for the land amounted to Rs. 51,000. He said that most of this money has already been spent in the day to day consumption needs of his large family, because they lost agricultural income all of a sudden. The family was provided one job which has gone to PR's eldest son. It is a labour grade job and the salary is Rs. 2,000 per month. Their house has not so far been acquired but it is going to be acquired soon. However, no compensation has yet been fixed and paid for it and a housing plot has also not been allowed to him so far.

PR was bitter about the present economic conditions of his people and said that even labour with the contractors was not available to the local people who were starving. Remembering the past, he said that Gharsani used to be a big village dominated by the Biyar and Brahmin. The Biyar were traditional healers. They used to collect herbs and roots which were used in treating various diseases. Since there were no forests any more, these medicines had become scarce and this source of income for Biyars as a caste has been lost. According to him the Biyar caste *panchayat* (*Tat*) has also disintegrated. He also complained of the change in the rituals, religious life and social practi-ces. His main concern was that marriages have become quite expensive now and the ritual worship of *Baigadeeh* and *Devi Sthal* have more or less been discontinued which was causing all kinds of difficulties for the people.

Case 9

BF Ahir is the Pradhan (headman) of village Khokhari, now living in Khokhari rehabilitation colony. He is quite an old man, aged about eighty years. He has a large family of seventeen persons. Originally he hailed from Bansi, where he had thirty acres of land in *'Varg-4'* category. The land was acquired by the NCL for the Bina coal fields project. BF stated that compensation was paid at the rate of Rs. 4,500 per acre by the railways for the land acquired to construct the main railway line while the NCL paid Rs. 7,000 per acre. This clearly shows that different authorities adopted different standards of valuation. BF got a compensation of Rs. 70,000 from the NCL and Rs. 12,000 from the railways. One of his son also got a job. He was also allotted a plot on Gadia site. He still retains some of this money. The rest has been spent.

BF stated that his old village Bansi had a large population of 'adivasis and other backward classes and a few families of Bania and Rajput'. Jobs have been given by NCL only to those people who had a large land holdings and hardly twenty persons from Bansi village have been provided jobs. In the Khokhari colony, about 50-60 families reside and more than half are Ahirs, about ten are tribals and the remaining are from other castes. Some of these people were provided plots in village Gadia but subsequently most of these allotments were cancelled and those people have been left without any house sites. He particularly referred to the Kharwar who had been given plots in Gadia but whose allotments were cancelled subsequently. Now some Kharwars have been given plots right by the side of submerged areas near hydel station. Their condition is pitiable because their houses get water logged and inundated during the rainy season and they lose their belongings. In spite of making repeated representation to the NCL nothing has been done to save them from misery.

Case 10

RA is a Panika and lives in Dibulganj rehabilitation colony near Anpara village. He has a relatively small family of six members. RA's original village was Kuldumry where he had some land. The village got submerged under Rihand reservoir and all the oustees moved to Dibulganj village. The Rihand authorities gave two acres land to each of those who had land at Kuldumry.

Dibulganj was subsequently acquired in 1981 by the UPSEB for Anpara Thermal Power Project. Thereafter the people moved to the rehabilitation colony Dibulganj. Dibulganj village had a population of about 3,000, out of which Chamar, Dharkar, Kharwar and Bania were nearly 80 per cent and the rest included Teli, Panika, Nai and Dhobi. The compensation given to these persons was @ Rs. 4,500 per acre of land and for their houses a plot of 60′ × 40′ size was given. However, there are some people who have not got plots till now. No facilities or money was provided for shifting. He also stated that they were forced to shift after their earlier resistance. In this connection some violence had also occurred in which even General Manager, Anpara was involved.

RA laments the conditions of Dibulganj rehabilitation colony very bitterly. He stated that apart from cash compensation and a plot nothing else was given to the PAPs though jobs and fully developed colonies were promised by the UPSEB. Hardly 15-20 persons among the oustees have been given jobs in Anpara and the displaced persons have also not been given any preference in other work opportunities such as contracts, shops, etc. by the project.

As regards facilities in the rehabilitation colony, it

was over-crowded with no facilities by way of proper roads, medical facilities, educational institution, community centre, etc. The colony lacks other amenities like drains and lights and even the pits and *nalas* in the colony have not been levelled. Therefore there is heavy water logging during the rainy season and a part of the colony becomes inaccessible. The plots were made by levelling the rocky lands and hillocks and therefore, it is not possible for the people themselves to improve the area. Digging of wells and ordinary hand pumps was not possible and drinking water facilities continued to remain quite inadequate. Dibulganj colony has accommodated almost all the oustees from 9-10 villages, Anpara, Audi, Dibulganj, Kudi, Parasi, Pipri, Sonwani, Belwadak, Kundabhant and Chittawar. With such a large number of oustees being rehabilitated at one place, wage-earning opportunities too have become scarce. The treatment meted out by the project officers was extremely bad. RA's impression was that the oustees from other projects in Sonbhadra had received a far better deal than those of UPSEB. RA also stated that the oustees had tried to organise themselves and fight for a better deal under the banner of an organisation called Visthapit Parishad. However, the project authorities refused to give any recognition to the Parishad for representing people's grievances and therefore the Parishad could not help them at all.

Case 11

RL belongs to the Jaiswal caste (Bania). He is literate and aged about sixtyfive. He has a large family of sixteen including three sons. His original village was Anpara and they were shifted to the Dibulganj rehabilitation colony. He stated that the compensation given by the UPSEB was @ Rs. 4,500 per acre. But this has not been paid fully as nearly 15 per cent of compensation is still to be received by the oustees. Moreover, the oustees from his village were also promised some ex-gratia payments to enable them to move but nothing has been paid so far. He stated that in the Anpara village the project authorities used a good deal of force. Bulldozers were used to remove some five-six families and there was violence in the process.

He also confirmed that labour work with contractors was not easily available in the area and the contractors paid only Rs. 20-25 per day instead of the full rate of about Rs. 40.

Case 12

Ms KM is a Panika and is educated upto Class VIII. Aged about twenty two years, she was married in village Vidar but she is now living in Dibulganj after displacement. She is teaching in the Balwadi school run by the Lokhit Manch, Navjeevan Vihar, Singrauli. The Balwadi is actually located at Pantsagar, Pipri. Her salary was Rs. 300 earlier but recently it has been raised to Rs. 400 which according to her is a meagre amount. She reported that the educational facilities in the area are very poor and therefore the Balwadi has even grown up children, both boys and girls, aged upto 8-9 years.

KM further stated that the Dibulganj rehabilitation colony lacks basic amenities like roads, electric connection, school, drainage and community centre. The project has employed not more than 25-30 persons. People have not been provided with any other rehabilitation facilities or relief. According to her the Panika have now become more aware about the modern world. Some Panika youth have set up a body known as Sun Club. The Club tries to organise outdoor games for young children. It is not a registered body.

Case 13

SB belongs to the Kharwar caste. He is sixty years of age with a large family of twenty-eight persons including four sons who are all married. He has been displaced twice. His original village was Kuldumry which was submerged in Rihand in the year 1961. As a result they moved to Mamuwar village two km. away where they had about five acres of land.

The second displacement came with their land in Mamuwar being acquired by the UPSEB. He got compensation @ Rs. 4,500 per acre and two plots (as his family was large) in the Dibulganj rehabilitation colony. SB says that most of this money has been spent. Beyond this, no other rehabilitation facility was provided by the UPSEB. None in the family has got a regular job and the able-bodied persons worked with the contractors at a low wage of Rs. 20-22 per day. He further stated that among the Kharwar, none got a job in Anpara project. There are about fifty Kharwar houses in the colony. He bitterly complained that the colony lacks all basic facilities including adequate supply of drinking water. 'This colony never received any attention from any political leader like M.L.A., etc.'

Case 14

Forty-five years old KP is a local leader. He is an educated Panika and lives in the Dibulganj rehabilitation colony. His family has been displaced twice. His original village was Kuldumry where his father had three and a half acres of land. When this village was submerged in Rihand, his father got a compensation of Rs. 1400. They moved to Anpara where they were given two and a half acres of land. This land was acquired by the UPSEB in 1981 and he got a compensation of Rs. 20,000, @ Rs. 4,500 per acre.

Recollecting his Anpara days, KP stated that the village had a population of 3,500. The important castes were Dharkar, Kharwar, Chamar and Bania. Other groups like Panika, Teli and Gond had twenty to forty houses each. There were a few houses of Brahmin, Dhobi and Nai also. All the people depended on agriculture and obtained subsidiary income from the forests. Preparation of catechu was also done by Kharwars. The Panika were previously weaving cloth when it was in good demand. Some people depended on making baskets and leaf-plates. The entire village was acquired by the UPSEB. Then some families moved away towards Sidhi (beyond Singrauli) and Sarguja in M.P. and Babhani (north-eastern portion of Sonbhadra).

Regarding the conditions of the Dibulganj rehabilitation colony and the treatment given to them by UPSEB, KP described it as *manmani* (high handedness). The main problem in the colony was lack of adequate drinking water. In fact drinking water was scarce almost throughout the year. Then, there were difficulties due to the lack of roads, drainage and cleaning, and water-logging. He said that there was a government junior high school near the colony but the project authorities had not provided any educational facility in this large colony itself. There was a ration shop but it seldom supplied rations and cards had not been issued to many. As regards electric light, medical facilities, community centre, etc. hardly anything had been done. He opined that the management of the colony and welfare of its residents was nobody's concern.

KP estimated that not more than twenty per cent of the people had got jobs. In fact no preference was given to the oustees by the UPSEB in providing jobs or work as contractors and the assignment of shops and kiosks, in spite of the opportunities which have come with the establishment of the project. He said that the contractors and shopkeepers in the project area were all outsiders and so were the employees.

The Dibulganj colony had people from nine villages acquired fully or partly by the project. These villages were Anpara, Ouri, Dibulganj, Pipri, Sonwani, Belwadah, Kundhant, Chittawar and Parasi (part). As this colony was large, they had formed an organisation—Visthapit

Parishad—for voicing their demands but the organisation could not take roots. However, people had now become more conscious and aware of their rights but still there was no response from the authorities. He concluded ironically that now 'people have come to know the meaning of *Mrityulok*'.

Case 15

HH is an old Baiga of about sixty years. He lives in the rehabilitation colony Gojahnwa set up by the Bijpur project. He has a large family of twenty-four. His original village was Gularia from where he and his father shifted in the year 1960 due to Rihand. There, they had fourteen acres of land which was in the name of HH's grandfather, who had died before the land was acquired. But no compensation for that land was given either to HH or to his father. The only compensation he got was Rs. 200 for the house. From Gularia the family moved to village Gojahnwa where they got seven acres of land for settling down.

The second displacement came in the year 1983 when NTPC acquired the entire village of Gojahnwa. He received compensation @ Rs. 7,500 per acre for three acres of land. The remaining four acres was *'Varg-4'* (forest) category land and therefore no compensation was paid for it. HH complains that no compensation has been given for his trees and his house. He is still living in the old house which is built on 'Varg-4' land. He expected that he would be given a plot of 60′ x 40′ when he shifted from this land. One of his three sons had been given a job in labour grade in the NTPC.

Talking of his old village, he narrated their past life vividly. With fourteen acres of land, their condition was quite good. Most of the things consumed in the family were grown by the family itself and only kerosene oil, salt and cloth had to be purchased. Certain produce from the forests were also available there. They could get fire-wood and timber for housing from the forests. In addition they were collecting other minor forest produce such as *anwala*, bamboo, and *bagai* grass which was used for making mats and weaving *charpai*.

The village had a number of caste groups living together. The *jajmani* system was practised. The Baiga were given land by the village people for performing ritual duties at the village *Baigadeeh*. Similarly a part of the farm produce was also given to the Nai, Pandit, Lohar and Dhobi, for their services. The Lohar or Agaria made iron tools and did *phargani* (repairs), the Nai did hair cut and shaving and a variety of duties on the occasion of marriage, *Chhati*, etc., the Chamars were drummers at the time of marriage and *puja*. The Baiga performed *matkorwa* and so on. However, the system has weakened with the loss of agricultural land. The Baiga *Panchayat* at Jawar and *Tat* levels were vigorous. This system had now ended and so have the religious practices. Some of the people from Gojahnwa moved away to Sarguja.

In the present colony, the problem of drinking water is acute. The colony has two wells and one hand-pump. The hand-pump remained out of order and wells dried up in summer. Electric connections were promised but not provided. There were no drains and roads. The colony had a primary school but no medical facility or community centre. There was a ration shop but most of the people did not have ration cards.

A regards wage labour, the contractors did not give work to the local people and when they did employ the local people they did not pay the fixed minimum wages. Instead, they paid Rs. 20 per day. Regular jobs have been given by the NTPC to about fifteen per cent of the oustees. The people of this colony had organised a body known as Kshetriya Vikas Yuva Samiti to agitate for their rights before the NTPC. Some of the people also sat on hunger strikes several times. However, they could not achieve anything. In his words—*abhi tak koi sunwai nahin hui* (so far no hearing has been given), "Our only demand was to get the minimum means of livelihood."

Case 16

Fifty years old SD is a Nai (barber). He is literate and has a family of fourteen including four sons, three daughters-in-law and their children. He lives in the rehabilitation colony Gojahwan. His original village was Mushwasi which was submerged in Rihand. There his father had fourteen acres of land. At the time of submergence compensation was paid to his father @ 30 times of land revenue. SD does not remember the exact amount of compensation and how it was utilised. From there they moved to Jarhan Bajandeeh where only seven acres of land was given to his father for rehabilitation. SD separated and shifted to Bijpur.

In Bijpur SD had purchased one bigha of land. The NTPC acquired it in 1983 and also his house. As compensation he had received only Rs. 5,000 for the house. Compensation for one bigha of land, the well he dug on the land and his trees had not been given to him so far. He could not indicate how much more compensation he had to get. He has been given a house plot of 60′ × 40′ but the plot has a rocky base and large rocks in front of it. Therefore he has not been able to build a proper house. No job has been provided to him.

In the old village the Brahmin and Koiri were important castes with about sixty houses each. Besides, there were a few houses of Rajput, Biyar and Panika. Chamar, Nai and Lohar had only one house each. All these people could not settle at one place and many of them moved away to Sarguja in M.P. or Babhani and Robertsganj in Sonbhadra. Emotionally he said that "the whole community has been disintegrated, there is no human link now with any one."

Case 17

HM is an illiterate Gond aged about fifty-five years. He

has a family of twelve which also includes his younger brother. He lives in the Bijpur rehabilitation colony. His original village was Bijpur where he had twenty acres of *sirdari* land. Others in the village were displaced due to Rihand while he was not affected. His first displacement came in the year 1982 when the entire land was acquired by the NTPC. He got a total compensation of Rs. 85,000 for land and house. He could not give a break-up of this amount. He stated that he did not get any compensation for about fifty trees (*Palas, Aam, Khair, Peepal, Mahua,* etc.) on his land and for a *kachcha* well that he had dug for irrigation. He has been given two plots in the colony and one job for his elder son. Though he was displaced in 1982 the job was provided only towards the end of 1986. Most of the compensation money had been spent in domestic consumption by them as agricultural income had stopped.

Remembering the conditions before displacement, HM said that cultivation was quite good on his land. Sugarcane was also grown by him and irrigation facility was available from the Rihand river. Originally the village was mainly of Gonds but as a result of the Rihand submergence some other caste groups had moved into the village. These included Teli, Kalwar (Jaiswal), Kewat, Lohar, etc. The forest around Bijpur was good and they could get fuel-wood and timber for houses as per their needs, and *Bagai* grass was available in plenty. He commented that due to the denudation of forests the rainfall in the area had decreased substantially. The diseases the Gonds suffered from were then cured with their traditional medicines. But now the same people had to go for expensive modern medicine. In the *Jajmani* system, Nai, Lohar, Dhobi and Baiga used to get grain from agriculturists twice a year. Gorait also used to get his due (*Kharwan*). He observed that in the Gond marriages previously, Pandit, Nai and Baiga were doing their customary duties and the Chamar used to play drums.

There was no dowry among the Gond but now demands for various modern household things like cycle, wrist watch, transistor, etc. are usually made by the groom's side. He felt that the *Birdari Panchayat* at *Jewar* and *Tat* levels had lost their authority or control.

In respect of the rehabilitation colony, he particularly mentioned the problem of drinking water. Besides, there was no electricity and proper roads or drainage within the colony. He said there was a government primary school for which the NTPC had built a good building but even in this school the teachers demanded money for admitting their children. No medical facility was available to them even though the colony had a population of more than a thousand. There was no ration shop and only some people had ration cards for the shop in another colony.

Case 18

BH belongs to the Mallah caste. He is more than fifty years old and has a family of eighteen including four sons, two daughters-in-law and five daughters. He lives in the Bijpur rehabilitation colony. He originally resided in Purwatola hamlet of Bijpur village where they had three acres of *Sirdari* land. His father got a compensation of Rs. 400 when their land was submerged in Rihand. Since he was a grown up person then he got two acres of land in Karitola as a Rihand oustee. His father got land separately.

About ten-eleven years ago the NTPC acquired the entire land in Karitola. His family was one of those who were forcibly removed and his house was bulldozed. The rate of compensation given was Rs. 7,700 per acre. The compensation he received was Rs. 15,000 for the land and Rs. 8,000 for the house. He said that he had received no compensation for his *pacca* well, half acre of land and 26 fruit-bearing and catechu trees on his land. Further, the family had received one plot of 60′ × 40′ and one of his sons had been given a labour grade job by the NTPC where he got a salary of Rs. 2,000 per month. BH emphatically stated that there was a lot of corruption in the payment of compensation and he had to pay the Amin, Lekhpal (revenue officials) and others in the tehsil nearly half of the compensation money as bribes.

Case 19

GN is Ahir by caste. He lives in the Bijpur rehabilitation colony. He is fifty years old and has a family of six including four daughters. His original village was Thanatola hamlet in Bijpur, where he had land. The land was submerged in the Rihand. He had received a compensation of Rs. 200 only. He also got three acres of land for his rehabilitation. In 1981 he was displaced for the second time as the NTPC acquired his land. This time he got a compensation of Rs. 4,000 (only for the land in his name) and Rs. 6,000 for his house. He said that he did not get any compensation whatsoever for the *'Varg-4'* land he was cultivating and fifteen trees, mostly fruit-bearing, on his land. He has been given one plot of 60′ × 40′ in the Bijpur rehabilitation colony where he has built a house. No job has been provided to him.

GN complained about drinking water, drainage and road facilities in the colony as well as about medical facilities. According to him "living amidst lack of basic facilities has become a part of our lives".

Case 20

Eighty-five years old DD is a Teli by caste and he is illiterate. He now lives in the Bijpur rehabilitation colony with his family of twenty-two members. His original village was Bijpur (plains) from whre he was displaced in 1960. He had twelve acres of *sirdari* land and twenty-five acres of *'Varg-4'* land at that time. He got a compensation of roughly about Rs. 2,000 for his entire holding and seven acres of land for rehabilitation in the year 1961-62.

His second displacement came when the NTPC acquired the area where they had shifted, on the upper side of Bijpur village. This acquisition came in the year 1981-82. By that time he was cultivating seven acres of land received as rehabilitation land and another twenty-two acres of *'Varg-4'* land. He received compensation only for the land in his name, amounting to Rs. 40,000 from the NTPC and five plots of 60′ × 40′ for himself, his sons and their grown-up children. It may be mentioned that DD has two middle aged sons and six grand-sons out of whom five are married. He pointed out that he was yet to get compensation for (i) his *'Varg-4'* land; (ii) well he had dug in the *sirdari* land; (iii) about fifty trees (14 mango, 14 guava, 2 lemon and another 20 of timber for building purposes), and (iv) three small *bandhi* which he had constructed on *'Varg-4'* land. Besides, one-third of the compensation fixed for his *sirdari* land had also been 'held back'. He said that he had been representing (*Bahut kaha suni aur likha padhi*) to the authorities for the balance of compensation and other claims for the last so many years without any result. Only one person in the family has been given a labour-grade job by the NTPC.

Case 21

RC belongs to the Gadaria caste. He is forty years old and lives in the rehabilitation colony Bijpur with his wife, one son and two daughters. His original village was Adhora, which was submerged in the Rihand reservoir. In that village he had five acres of land but he does not remember how much compensation was paid for that land, house, etc. because he was too young at that time. They settled in Nemna village where they were given two acres of land. He remembers that many of his neighbours in Adhora village moved to another village and not to Nemna. Later, RC shifted to Bijpur village where he 'purchased' three acres of *'Varg-4'* land.

RC was subsequently displaced when his land was acquired by the NTPC in 1981. He said that out of his three acres of land he received compensation only for two acres (Rs. 20,000) and for the house (Rs. 5000). No compensation has so far been paid to him for the trees and irrigation well he had on his agricultural land. He has also been provided with two plots of 60′ □ 40′ in the Bijpur rehabilitation colony. But in spite of all his efforts, the NTPC did not provide any job to him.

Case 22

Mrs. NM is fifty years old and belongs to Gadaria caste. She is a widow now living in Bijpur rehabilitation colony and has a family of four including one married son and one unmarried daughter. Three of her daughters have been married. She originally belonged to Mahuwaria hamlet of Bijpur village which was submerged in the Rihand reservour. She stated that her husband did not get any land for rehabilitation and the total cash compensation received by him was Rs. 500. They moved to village Dyodhar where they had about two and a half acres of *sirdari* land.

Their land in Dyodhar was acquired by the NTPC in the year 1981. She said that she had not received any compensation for that *sirdari* land so far. In Arauli village also she had two and a half acres of land and for that a compensation of Rs. 21,000 has been received by her. As regards residential plot, she has received two plots (60′ □ 40′) in the NTPC rehabilitation colony Bijpur. But no job has been provided to her sons. Now that they had no agricultural base, her sons supported the family by working as labourers with the contractors. She said that they earned only about Rs. 800 to Rs. 900 per month because work was not available for the entire month.

She concluded by emphatically saying that the NTPC people say that her *sirdari* land in Dyodhar was still in her possession but it was not a fact. In case of her Arauli land also the compensation does not cover twelve trees and one *pucca* well.

Case 23

RR, a Gond, is illiterate and about sixty years of age. He lives in the Bijpur rehabilitation colony with a family of nine, including three sons, two of whom are married. He was originally a resident of Bijpur itself. His land was not submerged in the Rihand. He was first displaced in the year 1982 when his six acres of *sirdari* land and four acres of *'Varg-4'* holding was acquired by the NTPC. He got a compensation of Rs. 45,000 for his *sirdari* land and Rs. 5,000 for his house. He has also been given two plots (60′ 40′) and one of his sons has been given a job in the labour grade with a salary of Rs. 2,000 per month. He had a *kachcha* well and about fifty trees including fruit-bearing trees on his land but no compensation has been given for that. Moreover, he has not received any compensation for his *'Varg-4'* land and one house which was in the name of his mother.

Remembering about his socio-economic conditions before displacement, he said that his land yielded three crops and thus they were quite well off. Besides, they also had access to the forests from where they got fuel-wood and minor forest produce. The hamlet was almost entirely of the Gond. Threfore, they had a vigorous community life. They had a *Devisthal* and *Baigadeeh* which was abondoned on displacement. He also stated that in the days of 'Singrauli Raj', the Gonds were very powerful. The *jajmani* system which benefited the Nai, Dhobi, Lohar, Baiga and Gorait was also practiced and the agriculturists gave them a regular fixed portion of their produce.

The present conditions were quite difficult as the people who lost their land ('their every thing') have not been provided jobs at all and they had to work with contractors at a low wage of Rs. 15-18 per day. Even this work was not available for the whole month. The living conditions in the colony were far from satisfactory.

Case 24

SR is an educated, forty years old Rajput. He lives in the Bijpur rehabilitation colony along with his family of eight members. He is an original resident of Bijpur village only a portion of which was submerged in the Rihand. He does not remember about the cash compensation received by his father. But they moved and settled in Dyodhar village where his father got seven acres of land for rehabilitation.

In 1982 NTPC acquired the land in Dyodhar. He said that compensation at the rate of Rs. 7,700 per acre was paid for his *sirdari* holdings. For housing he has got a plot of 60′ × 40′ but he has not been able to construct a house in the Bijpur rehabilitation colony because there is acute shortage of water in the colony. No job has been provided to him.

Speaking generally of the conditions, he made the following remarks :

(a) Though NTPC had put the oustees having agricultural land of one to two acres in the first priority category, hardly any oustee had been provided job since 1987.

(b) For getting small contracts and shops, the oustees were not given any priority/reservation. Outsiders got these benefits by describing themselves as oustees.

(c) Labour contractors generally paid half the fixed minimum wages. Since the oustees did not agree to this rate, the contractors preferred to bring their labour from outside.

(d) Compensation had been paid only for *sirdari* land and not *'Varg-4'* lands. Compensation for wells and trees had not been fixed properly. The compensation for trees does not take into

account the fruits they would have yielded or the cost of timber.

(e) There was extensive corruption in the actual payment of compensation because the system of payment through cheques, which was initially practiced, was given up subsequently. He said that compensations should be paid only by cheques in the presence of the community leaders.

(f) In the rehabilitation colony, hand pumps were mostly not in working order. Out of the wells, only two wells had water. In Dyodhar the piped water supply was inadequate. The taps ran for only twenty minutes, three times a day and one tap was shared by ten families or more. There was no facility of drinking water for cattle, no electric lights and no proper roads in the colony.

(g) Only a primary school had been provided. On the basis of the large population there should be at least four schools.

(h) Medical facilities were available only in a homeopathic dispensary. For allopathic medicines oustees had to go to the NTPC Hospital where they were generally discouraged and had to make payments.

(i) No ration cards had been issued to the oustees and there was no ration shop in the colony. In the NTPC there was a cooperative shop but the oustees could not get rations from there.

(j) A Panchayat Ghar had been provided in Dyodhar colony but not in Bijpur. There were no community centres.

(k) Even though the NTPC/Block organises inter-village sports every year, no facilities or play grounds have been provided by NTPC in the colony.

(*l*) The poorer sections among oustees—*Halwahas*, crop sharers, etc. had suffered acute difficulties as no rehabilitation benefits had gone to them. Even former land holders had no avenues of work. They had become 'like orphans'.

Case 25

LV aged about sixty-five belongs to Lohar caste (Vishwakarma). He narrated that generations back his ancestors came to the Singrauli state from Hardwar and settled in Bijpur area which was submerged in the Rihand reservoir. In the past a lot of patronage was given to the artisan communities like Lohar, Kumhar, Teli, etc. and his ancestors were given free land to settle in Bijpur by the then Raja Singrauli. In the beginning Bijpur was the capital of Singrauli state but internal feuds and occasional battles were common. Once a raja named Kunwar Saheb was injured by a bullet and then the capital was shifted to Gaharwar Gaon.

In his original village he had about twenty bighas of land and his family was pursuing the work of carpentry. Their land was taken by the local Scheduled Caste persons and one Kharwar family on share-cropping basis. In that village almost all the families, belonging to different communities, were agriculturists having some land and life was peaceful and prosperous. When the Rihand dam was constructed his village was submerged and people shifted to the high land of Bijpur. His family got a meagre compensation which he does not remember. But he got ten bighas of land in new Bijpur where he established his traditional work of carpentry. He informed that the government allotted land ranging 3½-10 bighas depending on the land ownership. But even landless people were given three bighas of land. The government provided one well and one school in such areas and the Soil Conservation Department provided help for levelling and *merbandhi* of the forest land. In due course of time people made this newly allotted land cultivable and resumed their normal life. In addition to this the land on the bank of Rihand was made available on *patta* to the cultivators. It yielded good crops when the water receded.

Then the area was taken up for acquisition by the NTPC and people were assured that they would be provided with water, electricity, house plots and jobs to one member of each family along with reasonable compensation. The process of uprooting them by demolishing their houses began. Their demand was land for land, since majority of oustees were agriculturists only and if one member of the family was given a job, others would have to look for a source of livelihood.

The district administration and NTPC officials said that land for land was not possible and the oustees could purchase land from the compensation money. It was decided on March 20, 1983 that the oustees would be given plots for house site as well as full payment of compensation. LV described with sarcasm what they had faced: labour work was available in plenty under contractors who were deployed for levelling and digging of land and they used to laugh at the hapless local people and their plight. This infuriated the people and they started an *andolan* (strike) for stopping the work. Then the district officials and the local Member of Parliament, etc. came to settle the issue and it was in their presence that the disbursement of compensation was initiated. But plots had not been earmarked or developed in the rehabilitation colony. It was a really precarious state, since it was the month of June when rains were expected. The authorities did not pay any heed and they were compelled to leave their houses along with their belongings during rains. It was a chaotic state of affairs as people were uprooted and no alternative sites for shelter was made available. The compensation for revenue lands was disbursed by the NTPC officers in the presence of the M.P., etc. and the NTPC people were so considerate then that the farmers who could not come on their own were provided vehicles and sometimes revenue stamps were also given by them for the receipts. But the land under forest i.e., '*Varg-4*' was not considered for compensation. On this issue, LV said, "local NGO Banwasi Sewa Ashram helped us and picked up five persons from each village to fight out the case in the Supreme Court. As a result of the judgement of the Court, one of its Commissioners visited the area for spot inspection and verification. Through him, some families got crop compensation for a period ranging between 1-3 years, about forty-five displaced families were given one job each in the project and twenty-two were provided some work on contract basis."

Describing the situation of the rehabilitation colony, LV was very critical and said that, "till 1988 the colony was in a very bad shape and when the then Energy Minister, Vasant Sathe, visited the area he ordered that piped water supply and electricity as well as roads, lanes, drains should be provided to cater to the need of all the houses. But till date it has not been done and only eighteen hand pumps, fourteen wells and a few roads (not touching Harijan and Adivasi houses) were made. Electric connection has not been given so far, though the police station just on the vicinity of the colony had been supplied with electricity. NTPC people said that their work was generation or production of electricity and not domestic connections which came under the purview of the U.P. State Electricity Board."

However, the NTPC started a training course of carpentry "for displaced youth belonging to Adivasis and Backward Classes." It was started on February 19, 1991, in the colony's primary school building. The trainees were not given any incentive in the form of stipend and they faced hardships. Later on it was decided that if the articles made by the trainees were accepted, they would get labour charge as incentive. LV was appointed as instructor of this training centre on payment of Rs. 50 per day. The training was for six months. In the beginning eighteen trainees joined the programme but at the closing stage of training only seven were left. Two courses were organised and ultimately on April 2, 1993, this centre was closed by the authorities and all the raw materials and finished articles were taken to their head office without any payment of labour to the trainees. This type of training if encouraged could have made the youth self employed but it lacked basic in-puts like allowances for the trainees. After completion of training, tools should have been given to the trainees to start their own work.

LV further said, "the loss of agriculture resulted in deterioration of inter-caste relations, since in agriculture artisans and labourers had a unique relationship. Now, with the change in time and attitude, people go for outwardly show; for example in good old days *Barats* were taken in a simple manner and local drums were used but now people think in terms of tent, band party and decoration which is quite costly. There was no custom of *Tilak* but it is becoming common now. The relations with the Adivasis were as labourers, share croppers and even Baiga was consulted in difficulties but the system has changed. Some old customs do continue in different forms but that does not fulfil the requirement of the *praja*" (people who render services).

Case 26

SH, aged about fifty, belongs to the Teli caste. His original village was Bijpur which was submerged in Rihand. There he had twelve bighas of agricultural land and his family members were doing cultivation. When this village was submerged his family shifted to high land of Bijpur. The amount of compensation they received was not known to him. His father got ten bighas of land and in due course of time another fifteen bighas were added. At the time of displacement by the NTPC in 1982-83 he lost all the twenty five bighas of land, his house, one well and thirteen trees. He has a large family consisting of twenty-two members including two brothers, parents and children. They got three plots for houses in the Bijpur colony. His younger brother got a job as a Store Keeper in the NTPC and gets about Rs. 2,000 per month. His father is quite old and remains at home. He himself undertook some work on contract basis from the NTPC and only a year back he was allotted a shop in the marketing centre of the colony where he had started a flour mill.

Most of the compensation money received by him was spent on construction of house and domestic consumption. The compensation for forest land under *'Varg-4'* had not been paid. He narrated that compensation was paid only after the local people resorted to agitation and on the intervention of the Collector and local M.P. in 1983 and only two-third compensation was paid at that time and one-third compensation had not been paid yet. According to him the NTPC and the District administration had played foul with them because the assurance at the time of ouster had not been fulfilled. A delegation of eight persons had met the then Revenue Minister in 1982 for the *'Varg-4'* land because most of the land in this area was of that category and the survey and settlement operations of the area in 1980-81 were questioned by the people. But the problem could not be solved. It was only after the Supreme Court judgement obtained through the efforts of the Banwasi Sewa Ashram that the matter had been settled. There were many opportunities for casual employment in the project through the contractors but these contractors preferred outside people as they did not want to pay the prescribed daily wage (Rs. 36.57 per day). They usually paid Rs. 18 to 20 per day. In this way the rules were not followed and local people were deprived of employment and other opportunities.

After the loss of land the age-old relationships with other castes, who used to work as share croppers, labourers, *halwaha*, etc. had undergone change. Now the service of the Baiga which was a must for starting agricultural operations or taking up any work in the forest or in different family rituals were no more needed. These days he is only called for worship of evil spirits occasionally and in marriage rituals. Nowadays, people had to purchase foodgrains from the market and a lot of money received as compensation had been spent over it. In the past the same people grew sufficient grains and the surplus was carried for sale to Mudisemar market on bullocks.

Regarding facilities in rehabilitation colony, SH said that the NTPC had agreed to construct overhead tank for supply of piped water to each house but so far it had not materialised. Only a few hand pumps and wells were provided. One homoeopathic dispensary was running which hardly fulfilled the needs of the colony. The NTPC hospital did not provide any facility to them except some concession on medical tests. The services of local midwife belonging to Chamar community were utilised at child birth and that was the only *jajmani* relationship which continued. Other *jajmani* relationships had been discontinued in the absence of agriculture.

Case 27

Fifty-five old BG belongs to the Ahir caste, living in the Bijpur rehabilitation colony. His family has eight members. His original village was Bijpur, where he had fifteen bighas of land. He recollected the past and said that in 1959-60 people of the area likely to submerge were repeatedly informed through the *Gram Pradhan* to leave their houses, but they could not imagine that water would rise so high as to inundate their villages, fifty miles away from Pipri where the dam was being built. A few families left but the majority stayed and faced the disaster. The oustees from Rihand were given cleared forest land ranging from 3¼ to 10 bighas but no jobs were provided. People settled in due course and the land was made cultivable. In Bijpur he got ten bighas as Rihand oustee and acquired another ten bighas of forest land. Besides this, there was the facility of getting of lands which became available after recession of the water of dam on temporary *Patta*. As such enough foodgrains were grown and surplus was marketed in nearby markets. In a way their life was happy and peaceful. However, the local people were not given any opportunity for pisci-culture and fishing in the dam.

Most of these lands were acquired from about 1982 for the NTPC and its levelling started from February 9, 1983. In this area there was no record of sale of land to help the assessment of market rate of land for compensation purposes. In a meeting the Collector, Mirzapur, took 1977 as the base year and decided that NTPC Shaktinagar rate of Rs. 4,500 per acre should be paid. This rate was not acceptable because of price rise since 1977. Their demand was for Rs. 10,000 per acre. In another meeting in which the Collector, local M.P. and M.L.A. also participated, the General Manager of NTPC did not agree to go beyond Rs. 6,000 per acre. Then on the intervention and efforts of Ram Pyare Panika M.P. the rate of Rs. 7,700 per acre was agreed upon. BG was paid two-third compensation for his ten bighas of revenue land and the balance was still pending. The compensation for *'Varg-4'* forest land had since been decided by the Supreme Court at Rs. 10,000 per acre after verification by the Commissioner appointed by the Court. BG's compensation for his ten bighas of *'Varg-4'* land was also pending this process.

BG got one house plot in the colony over which he constructed a four roomed house. His son did not get any employment though he was interviewed in 1987. Now, he was engaged in petty construction work which did not fulfil the requirements of the family. A major portion of the compensation was used for house construction and repayment of old loans. This colony had 485 plots (house) out of which about one-third were given to the Adivasis (Gond, Baiga, Panika) and Harijans, two-thirds to Teli and other backward castes like Lohar, Ahir and some to other castes. Commenting on the rehabilitation colony, he was of the view that every thing had been done half-heartedly, meaning thereby that the promises made by the authorities had not been translated into reality. Compensation money had been mostly spent on day-to-day household consump-tion, house construction and some had gone for motor-cycles, scooters and spent even on liquor. This money was not used for any alternative source of livelihood by the PAPs except for five or six persons who opened shops of foodgrains and articles of daily use. Commenting on the condition of the tribals he opined that this group was either cultivator or labourer with no ambitions for development. Hence compensation money was not profitably utilised by them.

According to him in the past payments for services were made in the form of grain and one *maund* (about 37 kg.) was given to the Lohar for a plough, one-fourth share of produce was given to the *halwaha*, and the *Purohit* and *Nai* who were also paid in the same fashion. Now, after the loss of agriculture, the old *jajmani* relations had broken up. These days, for services of midwife (*Chamarin*) at child birth payment was made either in cash or a *saree* was given. During *holi* a branch of *semal* tree was planted where *holi* fire was to be lighted. The Baiga used to do this ceremony, locally called *Sambat Katna*. He was still doing it and he was paid modestly for it.

Drinking water facility for animals was an urgent problem of the colony. The traditional folk dances like Karma were on decline. A Kshetriya Sangharsh Yuva Samiti was formed to fight for their rights. In 1991 its worker sat on a *dharna* for 49 days. Vijay Singh, the then

M.L.A. arranged a meeting with NTPC officials for providing labour at approved rates. They were assured of getting work with contractors at approved rate, but hardly fifteen persons got the work with big contractors. BG was of the view that contractors should be ordered to recruit displaced persons first and then outsiders should be employed, but nobody bothers.

Case 28

SS is a Chamar and he is sixty-two years old. He lives in the Bijpur rehabilitation colony. His original village was in old Bijpur where he had ten acres of land and he was cultivating it. His family got a meagre compensation for displacement and thirteen bighas of uneven land in highland Bijpur. According to him life in the past was tension free as all members including women were engaged in cultivation; children were engaged in grazing and collection of forest produce. In due course the newly allotted land was made fit for cultivation and its produce was sufficient for his family. Subsidiary income from the traditional occupation of *dai* by Chamar women folk was also there. Rihand displacement was not remembered much as his parents were alive but the displacement caused due to NTPC was bad for him and his caste members. His land and house, etc. were acquired without any place for settlement and the present plot was given only in 1986. So he had to remain on the outskirts of the project in semi-built or temporary shade along with his family members. He got Rs. 70,000 as compensation for his land, house, etc. from the project. He had four sons, three of them married and the youngest one was studying in Adarsh Vidyalaya. His two daughters were married. He came to the present colony three years back and constructed his house on the plot spending about Rs. 15,000 from the compensation money. He was advised to keep the money in bank and he did it accordingly. Out of this money almost all except Rs. 10,000 had been spent on household consumption, marriages and house construction. One of his sons got employment in the project at a salary of Rs. 2,000 per month. Others were without any assured employment and were engaged as daily labour. His wife continued with the *dai's* work but the other women of the family were not interested in this type of work.

According to him NTPC had done a lot of harm to them by depriving them of their agriculture and providing no work. When reminded about the job given by NTPC to one of his sons, he said "it was all right but that boy became a stranger to us with a separate establishment." Only four or five persons could get service from the twelve Chamar families who were displaced. Their condition was not good, only seven got plots and four families were still staying on the outskirts of Bijpur. In the past "Baiga of the village had many important jobs to do for the village and its different castes for which he used to get grains but now his role has diminished."

The colony has roads, school, handpumps and wells. At present SS along with his family was living in a temporary structure in a vacant area and has given his two-room apartment on rent. His general complaint was that the displaced youth had not been provided with any assured nature of work and they were indulging in habits of consuming liquor and gambling. Adivasis' condition was no better. Some persons of Jaiswal and Teli castes had invested in transport business because they got more money by way of compensation and knew the tricks of business. Others did not know how to make better use of money.

Case 29

LJ aged about fifty-five years is a Chamar by caste and lives in Chilkadand after the displacement. He narrated that his original village was Khairwa, adjacent to the fort of Raja of Singrauli where their family was living in peace and prosperity, having more than thirty bighas of agricultural land. The land revenue was Rs. 2 per *bigha*. After the submergence of his original village he got about Rs. 3,300 as compensation of land, house and well, and settled in Kota village where his family purchased ten bighas of land. The other members of his caste went to Bijpur area. His family got only seven bighas of land at Nimyadand in lieu of submergence in Rihand dam.

In 1976, his land at Kota village was acquired by the NTPC and he got compensation of Rs. 12,000 for only four bighas of land whereas his father got a compensation of Rs. 16,000 for land and Rs. 20,000 for house, well, trees, etc. In Nimiyadand he had a house and some land for agriculture also. Under rehabilitative measures he got two plots at Chilkadand and two plots at Nimiyadand. He got employment in NTPC on muster-roll basis with a salary of Rs. 2,200 per month. His two sons were also working in the project.

LJ said that his father died four years ago, his mother lives at Nimiyadand and two sons were looking after agriculture. One son is studying in class eighth. He informed that employment has been provided by the NTPC only to those who had one acre or more of land. His economic position was sound, as he had a double storeyed house on two plots at Chilkadand, a well inside the house, three buffaloes and one Ambassador car. Among Scheduled Castes, his family was economically well off and commanded respect in the locality. He showed his house where a number of cracks on the walls were caused by the blasting and said no household items could be put on the raised platform and many times metallic utensils fell from any place above the ground level. There was always danger to life and property.

LJ narrated a number of problems being faced by the families living in Chilkadand, the most important ones were as follows :—

(*a*) Electric connections for domestic use were not

provided.

(*b*) The railway track near the colony was posing danger for the life of animals and human beings.

(*c*) The cattle were not safe and these were stolen with the connivance of police and sold in Madhya Pradesh.

(*d*) Apart from a homoeopathic dispensary, no medical facility was made available.

(*e*) Blastings by the NCL was also a menace to the locality and residents.

Case 30

AK is a young man of thirty-two years. He is a Panika. He narated his experience of displacement. His late father and other members of the family were residing in village Yogi-Chaura and had one bigha of agriculture land, one big house and five cows and two bullocks. In 1981 his family was displaced by the NTPC and at that time he was studying in Junior High School at Dudhi. When he returned to his house he found his family members under a tree with household goods. He had three brothers and three sisters and they got two plots at Kharia, 50′ × 30′ each. The project did not provide any employment. His elder brother got a government job in U.P. Secretariat and he stayed at Lucknow with his family. AK with his wife, two children and mother lives at Kharia. At the time of displacement, Rs. 400 were received as compensation. He studied upto Intermediate and did *'A'* Grade training of Wireman from I.T.I., Lucknow. He was the Joint Secretary of an organisation established in 1991 named as Udvasit Berojgar Sahkari Shram Samvida Samiti.

AK said that about 1800 families had been displaced on account of the NTPC Project and against it only 400 persons could get employment in the project. The unabsorbed families met the then Union Power Minister,

Vasant Sathe when he visited the area. The minister advised them that as long as they were not provided jobs they should form a labour cooperative society and obtain contracts form the project. The minister had further assured them that the uprooted families whose land, house, etc. had been acquired and who did not get any type of employment, would be given Rs. 100 per month each as unemployment allowance. But this never materialised. Two months later, the then Prime Minister, Rajeev Gandhi visited the area and he too assured them in a public meeting that whatever Sathe had declared must be fulfilled. These assurances did not find favour with the authorities and the condition of unemployed youth continues to be pitiable.

The Samiti referred to above could get contract for two types of works in NTPC for one year in which seventy-four persons got daily wage at the rate of Rs. 38.57. Their Samiti could not afford to compete with moneyed contractors and lost its contract. The NTPC must give relaxation to the Samiti and only then the unemployed persons can get a source of livelihood.

Case 31

RK is fifty-one years old, belonging to the Thakur caste and resides in village Chetwa. He had studied upto middle (VIII) standard in 1956 and is a social worker. He along with his family members was living in village Modra which was submerged in Rihand lake in 1960. He received 6¼ bigha of cleared forest land at Chetwa but he moved to village Katauli in Sidhi district of M.P. and the land at Chetwa was looked after by another person of Chetwa. He used to visit this place 2-3 times a year. His brothers were still living in M.P. where too they had land but he finally shifted to Chetwa in 1974. Out of his five sons and three daughters, one daughter and two sons were married, his son-in-law was working in Jayant Coalfields of NCL in M.P. and two of his sons were looking after agriculture and dairy. Now in the village he owned about twenty bighas of land, some belonged to his uncle and some was purchased by him. He said that he had donated a part of the land to the Banvasi Sewa Ashram. He had a plantation of eucalyptus *sheesham*, and bamboo on ten acres of land adjacent to the Ashram. He had a tractor and a tube well of his own. He had five buffaloes and two Jersey cows and, on an average, got 35 litres of milk per day. He supplied milk to the project on contract basis. The cultivation was done through local labour for which he paid Rs. 15 per day to male and Rs. 12 per day to female labourers.

Though RK had not been affected by the NTPC so far, but being a social worker and educated he had taken all possible benefits like supplying vegetable and milk to the NTPC project. He said that the criteria for employment in the project was loss of land and the families who lost two acres or more land were provided employment. In rehabilitation colonies No. 1 and No. 2, about 600 plots of the size of 60′ × 40′ were earmarked for the displaced families. According to RK, the Adivasis were about 20 per cent of the affected families, and on an average Rs. 30,000 each was received by them as compensation. A Jaiswal family (four brothers) got Rs. 8 lacs as compensation. But since the displaced families were mostly illiterate and ignorant they could not utilize the money in a profitable manner. A few had invested in petty business but when outside Banias came their business was ruined. By and large people utilised the money for household consumption. In some families the young boys purchased motor-cycles and scooters. There should have been some programme for the displaced families like poultry, vegetable growing, milk production, etc. which were items of daily consumption by a large number of employees of the project, but nothing had been thought of in this direction and the people were left to decide their future themselves. The contract work in the project which was mainly the supply of coal, bricks, sanitation, plantation, etc. generally went to outsiders as the officials of the project preferred to oblige their kith and kin. Local labour is preferred only on paper but not encouraged because they demanded the minimum wage (Rs. 36.57 per day) whereas outside labour would gladly accept Rs. 25 per day.

Discussion

A holistic picture of reality emerges from these cases. The projects were established one after another. But no where do we come across any local participation before the onset of any project or any advance preparation of the people to enable them to derive benefits from the ensuing construction and production activities (Sharma 1975). The projects displaced the people once, twice, and in some cases four times. A few people got jobs, some others started a business, still some others got into occupations which were earlier unknown to them but it was all sporadic. Besides these, many other dimensions came into focus with regard to their new social life. When one goes through the above cases objectively, the following issues emerge :

(a) The projects though executed with all gracious intentions of development, both at the community level as well as individual level, were least helpful to the displaced people. The benefits of even the products of the projects were not given to the oustees. For example HC lamented that lamp-posts had been erected but the colony is dark. Even the colonies adjacent to the power project were dark.

(b) The local people were not taken into confidence before the onset of any project. In most of the areas the news of the establishment of the projects and consequent displacement came as a nightmare to the people. Hence there was no

question of any local participation.

(c) Disparity at the level of compensation packages to the oustees is clearly visible.

(d) A hierarchical structure emerged at two levels : *(i)* 'we and they', that is to say 'we' are the oustees and 'they' are the 'powerful project wala' (project authorities) and *sarkar* (government), and *(ii)* an internal stratification that emerged within the oustees themselves—some of them got good cash compensation and developed a few entrepreneurial endeavours whereas most failed to utilise the money or got meagre compensation, thus resulting into new rich and poor categories. The first category comprised of emigrants to the area some of whom came first before the projects and managed to get lands recorded in their names.

(e) Lack of a human and democratic approach on the part of authorities while displacing people was evident in all projects. Rather than persuade the people through a 'dialogue', and providing them with the necessary wherewithal, coercive measures were adopted to evacuate them, in quite a few cases. Their houses have been bulldozed.

(f) People's protest—whether lawful or unlawful was not taken into cognizance and either they were overlooked or they were ruthlessly suppressed.

(g) All displacements and the consequent rehabilitation schemes and compensation packages present chaotic scenes. As RM said, "we knew earlier that *'Sarkar'* is installing the project for which they had surveyed the area. I shifted but others did not and had to suffer suddenly when, over night, water ran into their houses." Here RM's conformist approach of abiding by the government's orders does not necessarily mean that he shifted with all willingness. Rather it was done due to RM's sense of awe, over the hegemonic control by the state. Regarding compensation in terms of cash or providing house plots, jobs, many odd incidents have occurred. Some oustees were given house plots immediately, some others got it after a lot of persuasion and still others never got it. People wanted to work as labourers in the project sites. Minimum wages were never paid and the contractors employed their own people since they were satisfied with a lower wage. One incident worth mentioning shows the fulfilment of sadistic pleasure : at NCL, when the oustees were working as labourers with the contractors, the latter used to laugh at the oustees. In another case (CK), one fails to think logically about the correlation between getting a job and family planning! People ultimately had to remain contented with whatever compensation they got. The age old colonial concept of *praja* being at the 'mercy of officials' does not seem to have changed even after 50 years of independence.

(h) Heterogeneity among communities deepened due to the displacements. Earlier people belonging to different castes and tribes living together in the same village had evolved a socio-economic bond chiefly through *jajmani* and other links, which have been completely disrupted after displacement. In rehabilitated villages they encountered strangers since oustees from different villages were settled in one colony. Thus the strength of socio-cultural bond weakened.

(i) The entire socio-cultural fabric of the villages

has been lost due to displacement. The religious practices have been discontinued due to the loss of forest land as well as agricultural land. *Baiga Deeh* is worshipped no more. Kin groups have dispersed and the most trusted cooperation from kins are no more there during exigencies. Marriage customs have changed. Instead of bride price now tribals have started practising dowry system. This is a clear indication of Hinduization. The *panchayat tat* is no more there. People now truly suffer from a 'culture shock'.

(j) Mode of production has changed drastically. The age old agricultural mode of production has been changed with the industrial set-up. But there is no clearcut mode of production and people no more get medicinal herbs to cure themselves, from forests and Baiga does not go to cure others. For domestic consumption they need money. New avenues of consumerism have come up. The money economy has barged into their traditional set-up.

(k) Overall, there has been no rehabilitation policy followed in these areas which is also the all-India situation. The lack of policy resulted in the deteriorating conditions for the oustees who once lived on their own and had a 'life of contentment and happiness.'

To conclude, it may be observed that the well organised village communities have been fragmented and what has come about is 'tearing apart of the social fabric' (Cernia 1991). Earlier, the tribes and castes used to live together, having achieved a *modus vivendi* and some symbiosis. They were part of a living social organisation and a cohesive structure of economic and social relations. Now, such communities have largely disappeared from the affected areas as no rehabilitations were planned for the communities as such. The social structure of individual tribal communities is also under serious threat, having been disturbed by the relocation of its constituents at far flung places. Their organisation and its socio-economic linkages are presently in a state of flux, even trauma, and it will take a long time for them to assume even atrophied coherence.

7

EMERGENCE OF LEADERSHIP

SOME aspects of village and community leadership in the area have been discussed earlier in this study. Broadly speaking, leadership in the tribal areas predominantly inhabited by one or two tribal communities is found to be generally strong and well organised and buttressed with the traditional leadership conventions and its supportive institutions such as youth dormitories. Singh (1982) in his study of tribal movements found that tribal unrest assumes an organised character only among the large, homogeneous land owning tribal communities who have a relatively strong economic base. In a multi-ethnic community, characterised by economic interdependence among different groups a movement, particularly the one connected with economic issues, takes a different course of development. But in an area inhabited by a large number of tribal groups mixed with a substantial proportion of emigrant non-tribal population leadership in the sphere of economy and secular interests of the community is found to be segmentalised, diffused and oft-changing. Here, the growth of any cohesive leadership is also hampered by a lack of education and awareness, especially among the tribal groups, and clash of tribe/caste interests. No effective movements supporting or agitating for any common cause can grow out of such a matrix. Such a vacuum in leadership is often filled up by the entry of social or political workers or other functionaries coming from outside, often linked with some regional or national movements usually aiming at economic and social reforms. Some recent examples are the Naxalite cadres in Andhra Pradesh (Adhikary and Bhattacharya 1982) and M.P., Sarvodaya workers in the Narmada Bachao Andolan and Chipko elements in the Tehri agitation.

Voluntarism draws its inspiration from the concept of social justice and it has been an integral part of the socio-political and cultural life of our people since long. In fact non-governmental initiatives in the course of our non-violent struggle for freedom helped largely in creating mass awareness. Gandhiji's call for constructive work laid the foundation for that struggle, in the early twenties through the creation of a large number of organisations for social action and service. In the field of tribal welfare his lieutenant A.V. Thakkar took the initiative to create organisations in different parts of the country. Soon after independence Vinoba Bhave took up rural reconstruction work in tribal and backward areas through his wide spread and wide spectrum movement for Bhoodan, Gramdan, Sarvodaya and Anantyodaya. It was seen that in the Sonbhadra area also the innate vacuum in leadership and the state of inertia was changed through the positive role of voluntary work taken up by people having link with the Gandhian plans of reconstruction and Sarvodaya. The approach and role of the few NGOs found active in the area may now be discussed.

Banwasi Seva Ashram, Gobindpur

The tribal areas of Sonbhadra have been drought prone areas. However, when the forests were in plenty the distress caused by drought conditions was not always very acute. The year 1952-54 saw a severe drought and the government took up relief measures. G.B. Pant, the then Chief Minister of U.P., had visited the area and in the words of Prembhai, the most prominent social worker in the area, he was seen actually in tears in the Dudhi dak bungalow over the prevailing conditions. He had then suggested that a non-government organisation should be set up for social services and rural reconstruction in the area. As a result, the Banwasi Seva Ashram was established in 1956 by some freedom fighters and reputed Gandhian workers of the State for the amelioration of the tribals and other poor communities living south of the Kaimur. Pant himself was one of its founders and Vichitra Narayan Sharma, 95 years old veteran Gandhian, has been its Chairman from the beginning. The Ashram covers about 400 tribal villages scattered over a forested, hilly area with a recurring history of drought and famine. Among the early activities of the Ashram were a school for tribal children, training in spinning and weaving and Bhoodan and Gramdan work.

In 1964-65 again there were acute famine conditions and a drought relief committee visited the area. Prem Bhai, a Sarvodaya worker, was a member of this committee and he was so much moved by the conditions that he decided to stay on in the Banwasi Seva Ashram itself and take up its work. This was in fact the real beginning of not only social services but also a new leadership to tackle the problems of the area. Prem Bhai started planning for more enduring work towards self sufficiency and self reliance in the villages. He drew up the AGRINDUS Project for the agro-industrial development. Firstly, attention was given to land development, ravine reclamation, bunding, and rain water harvesting with its management for irrigation. Introducing a variety of new crops of paddy, wheat, vegetables, fodder and fruit orchards, to eliminate drought and food deficit was the other step. Prembhai's wife, a medical doctor simultaneously planned for a community health and family welfare programme.

The third activity taken up by the Ashram was education and literacy. In 1967 literacy was only seven to nine per cent in these villages. With the help of the Literacy House, Lucknow, one hundred literacy centres and circulating libraries were set up in 1968. Educational activities of the Ashram have since grown to include eight primary schools, 160 non-formal education centres for working children, 100 adult education centres and training facilities in twenty-two vocations. But the core of the educational activities is the awareness building, campaigns for the conservation and development of environment and forests, elimination of alcoholism and other unhealthy traditions like untouchability, child marriage, dowry, etc. In mid 70s the Ashram initiated some other activities related to rural reconstruction on the Gandhian lines as well and a project known as the Rural Entitlement and Rural Support Services. While conducting village surveys for the latter project the Ashram workers came face to face with problems of debt bondage, the question of title for tribal lands, discussed in detail elsewhere, and various dimensions of displacement caused by the projects which had started coming up. The strategy and approach of the Ashram, undoubtedly modelled on the Gandhian and Sarvodaya lines included: (i) study/survey of the problem to highlight the facts and justify the cause of the tribals; (ii) creating public awareness about the facts and issues; (iii) creating consciousness in the tribal population affected; (iv) exploring the legal and constitutional methods available to the tribals by (a) approaching the bureaucracy and the State Government for redressal, and (b) by appealing to the judiciary, the Supreme Court, to uphold and enforce the legal rights of the tribals to their land, occupations and environment; (v) preparing the affected tribal populations for direct action and its consequences; and (vi) launching non-violent direct action. This approach has achieved a significant order from the Supreme Court upholding the right of the tribals to their lands and outlining modalities and a machinery for the redressal of their grievances. Since the work of the Ashram was mainly in the Bijpur area its encounter with the plight of the PAPs came when the NTPC started displacing the villagers for the Rihand-Bijpur thermal power project in February 1983. The question of compensation to be paid to the displaced people was closely interlinked with their titles over the land for which the Ashram had been fighting.

Thus, we find that by the close of the 70s Prembhai and his band of workers had been able to establish themselves in the area and win peoples' confidence. They were therefore in a position to organise a "non-institutionalised collective action' (Shah 1990) to grapple with the problem of land rights, the most basic need of the people, particularly the tribals. Prem Bhai passed away recently and now the Ashram is being managed by his wife.

Srajan Lokhit Samiti, Vindhaya Nagar

This is the other important NGO involved basically with the problems of the PAPs. However its headquarters are at Singrauli in Sidhi district of Madhya Pradesh and it, therefore, works most among the PAPs of NTPC, Vindhaya Nagar and NCL units in Madhya Pradesh. Awadesh who heads this organisation is a younger person who got his initiation through the Samagra Kranti movement launched by Jayprakash Narayan in the pre-emergency days. Thereafter he became associated with Setu an organisation based in Delhi which had its centres in many areas of Bihar, M.P., and Maharashtra, both tribal and non-tribal, where people were facing problems related to land, environment, etc. However, Setu was mainly confining itself to organising surveys, seminars and studies highlighting the problems and, by-and large, was not taking up any lead in organised agitations. Awadesh came to Singrauli area in connection with a survey and after acquainting himself with the conditions decided to set up a base there. The Samiti was registered in 1980 and started its work in 1983, primarily in the realm of studying and analysing the problems of the PAPs in the Singrauli area (both on M.P. and U.P. sides). In July 1984, it organised a seminar on these problems in which prominent media persons, activists and the tribal leaders of the area participated. Their publication, *Vikas Ki Keemat* (Setu 1985) was the outcome of this seminar. Since then the Samiti has been active mainly in the field of studies, workshops, etc. relating to the tribal problems and spreading education among them.

Their other activities include opening of several Balwadis for the children of PAPs, organisation of gram mandals, public libraries and a public awareness (*Janchetan*) campaign. Awadhesh, in the course of discussions, frankly admitted that the Samiti had not been as vocal and active as it should have been. He said that there were a large number of people interested in the problems of the tribal PAPs but the Samiti itself had not been able to provide the necessary feedback to them so that they could address themselves more effectively to this area. He claimed that for the 90s he had prepared a more comprehensive programme for the Samiti. They planned to concentrate on ecological regeneration together with agricultural development which would directly benefit the PAPs. The Samiti however does not seem to be having a wide base of grassroot workers which is the strength of the Banwasi Seva Ashram.

The Servants of India Society, Mirzapur Branch

The Servants of India Society, Pune was founded by Gokhale. Its U.P. branch was set up by Hridaya Nath Kunjru and Rama Shanker Mishra more than fifty years back and started work in the old Mirzapur district. The strength of the Society lies in its band of life members who dedicate their entire life to the Society's work. They are provided financial support for their personal needs by the Society. The Society now has two sub-branches in

U.P., one at Bazpur (Nainital district) carrying out schemes for the Scheduled Tribes in the Tarai and Hill areas while the second sub-branch is at Mirzapur. The organisation has, however, kept itself confined to educational and women welfare work on a limited scale even though it is the oldest organisation in this area with centres located in some of the most interior places. Had they addressed themselves to the cause of displaced persons they could have commanded a ready rapport and people's confidence. Presently the activities of the Society include running primary and higher schools, hostels for tribal boys and girls and women welfare centres with government grants.

Besides these there are a couple of other organisations whose work has remained confined to small pockets of the rehabilitation area. The representatives of these organisations and our informants generally comp-lained that the project authorities and the administration did not allow the organisations to take roots. In fact they did everything to discourage the organisations.

Discussion

The dynamics of a movement for land right and how the right of the PAPs became a part of it may now be traced briefly. After the Ashram workers encountered it in the course of their work for the reconstruction of village economy—the important phases of the Ashram's moves were as below :

(i) Prembhai and his team, including a sociologist with a law degree, took up a survey of five villages to find out the legal and administrative aspects of the land question.

(ii) Based on this detailed documentation of the situation, the Ashram decided to file a public interest petition before the Supreme Court. Thus they took recourse to an 'institutionalised

option' (Shah 1990) as their first choice. The Supreme Court issued an interim order in July 1982 banning eviction of the cultivators by the Forest Department and laying down a three months schedule for survey, settlement operations and setting up of a high power body by the State Government to settle all disputes on the spot.

(iii) The Government of U.P. then sought more time for survey and settlement and appointed a High Level Committee (Maheshwar Prasad Committee) to examine the status of the land records. The Committee made its report in December 1983 with findings seen as quite favourable to the Ashram's stand. But the State Government started dithering and procrastinating measures to implement the Committee's recommendations.

(iv) The tribals became restive as their expectations which rose after the Supreme Court order were not fulfilled and an environment leading to some 'non-institutionalised collective action' (Shah 1990) was thereby created. A front for the movement, known as the Bhumi Haqdari Morcha was created with representatives from nearly 400 villages of the area. Pratap Bhai became the Morcha Convenor and he started a publicity campaign through the local and national press, and also started educating the people in general about the situation and their demands. An eleven page memorandum was submitted to the State Government and a delegation also went to Lucknow to meet the Chief Minister and Revenue Minister and press for an early implementation of the Maheshwar Prasad Committee's recommendations.

(v) In the meantime work on the NTPC's Bijpur

plant was started in February 1983. The project and district authorities started using coercive pressures to oust the villagers from areas noti-fied for acquisition without actually paying them any compensation or giving facilities to enable them to shift and settle elsewhere, as they had done in case of the earlier NTPC project. This added to the discontent and a confluence of the twin problems—rights over land and for rehabilitation which were closely interlinked legally and on the ground. While pockets of resistance built up, hopes for institutional relief through the Supreme Court were dashed mainly due to the legal tangles created by the State Government.

(vi) Significantly, the rehabilitation and displacement issues were brought before the Supreme Court by the NTPC itself. As the lands, rights for which were being adjudicated by the apex court, included areas required by the NTPC and the former had in its interim order imposed a state of *status quo-ante* on their possession, the NTPC got itself impleaded as a party. The NTPC prayed that as the completion of the project was a time bound programme the land earmarked for it be made free from the prohibitive directions. The Court disposed of the matter finally in February 1992.

(vii) The Morcha's second initiative of 'institution-alised action', viz. petitioning the government and meetings with the Chief Minister did not elicit a positive and sympathetic response from the government. Therefore they resolved to take up a road blockade from the midnight of October 1, 1986 onwards to force the issue. The district administration used overwhelming force to remove the blockade but this step succeeded in focussing the attention of the media and the higher authorities to the demands and simultaneously the matter was brought to the notice of the Supreme Court. The local authorities pointedly tried to impute ulterior motives to Prembhai and his workers. They alleged that he was organising the agitation in order to divert attention from the inquiries in the Ashram's affairs by the Kudal Commission. This Commi-ssion was appointed by the Government of India in 1977-78 to enquire into the financial management of the Gandhi Smarak Nidhi and its associate organisations. The authorities also alleged that Prembhai was adopting a Naxalite approach to create law and order problems.

(viii) At this stage an organization called the Chhetriya Visthapit Samiti was also set up in the Bijpur area under the Ashram's initiative. The attempt of the NTPC authorities to get the acquired villages vacated even before any arrangements had been made for rehabilitation, etc. was thwarted through the Samiti's *Bandh*. The *Bandh* succeeded in stopping the construction work for the Bijpur project for several days in May, 1983 and ended when the project authorities expedited work in the colonies and payment of compensation.

The Ashram's approach to the problem thus seems to have started with 'institutionalised action', both before the judiciary and the government. It was subsequently changed to 'non-institutionalised collective action of protest and agitation'. However the agitation was never violent and its idiom was Gandhian, obviously because the leadership was of Sarvodaya workers though the local officials tried to discredit it by calling it a Naxalite move. Eventually the agitation succeeded when the Supreme Court passed comprehensive orders on the twin issues of land rights and rehabilitation. The orders of the apex court also more than vindicated Prembhai's own role and leadership as he was appointed a Commissioner of the Supreme Court to inquire into the implementation of the Court's orders and report to the Court from time to time. In this capacity Prembhai submitted a number of reports, *inter alia*, covering the progress of rehabilitation of the Bijpur oustees.

It is also, however, noticed that the role of the Ashram has been largely confined to the Bijpur project area in so far as the problems of PAPs are concerned. Prembhai has not organised any movement for the oustees of the NTPC's Shakti Nagar Project or UPSEB's Anpara project and the three NCL projects in Sonbhadra. The reason for this limitation seems to be that Prembhai was able to create a movement for land rights around the year 1981-82 and assume its pre-eminent leadership. The Shakti Nagar and Anpara displacements had occurred earlier and, moreover, the areas affected by these projects as well as the NCL projects were at a distance from the tract which had come under the influence of the Ashram. Even though Prembhai could obtain a very favourable order in respect of the rehabilitation measures for the Bijpur oustees in 1992 he had started feeling worried about its proper implementation when we met him a year later. He was quite critical of the failure of the project authorities on several counts such as infrastructural facilities in the colonies, provision of employment, and training for alternative skills, etc. Perhaps this adverse ground reality deterred him from making any plans for the other areas.

The experience of the leaders of the movements has been that the project authorities take to a variety of coercive or extra-legal measures to ensure that either the movements or agitations, even peaceful ones, do not materialise or if they do some how assume shape, they fail in their aims. As Awadesh pointed out, the first part of this strategy is to question the very *locus standi* of the leaders or the spokesmen of the organisation representing the oustees. Generally, the protests are handled by the people who deal with labour and personnel problems in the project administration who, in keeping with their usual approach in that area, initially take the stand that the NGO in question had not been 'recognised' by the project to speak or agitate on behalf of the oustees. As if the oustees were also a part of the project staff or labour and needed an 'officially recognised union' to speak for them. In this way the project authorities at first try to maintain their inaccessibility and lack of transparency. Later on if the protest is successful in assuming a concrete agitational form such as some strong procession, demons-tration, *dharna, anshan*, etc. the project's attitude is to ignore it in every way or to deny all justification for it and its demands through inspired compaigns in the media. Further, if inspite of such initial efforts, the protest gets established, continuous or recurring, the senior level officers enter the picture and initiate talks for a settlement, usually in a 'deliberate hurry'. When such negotiations are set afoot, the momentum of the agitation gets immediately dissipated. Then the officers often delay any finalisation of the negotiations by subterfuges like the need for consulting the higher authorities or obtaining legal opinions. This further delay in their making any commitments to the agitators starts telling upon the agitation, specially because these people are poor, sustaining themselves on daily labour and cannot, therefore, continue with days-long agitation. Furthermore, even when such an agitation succeeds in getting some demands conceded and a settlement is reached the project authorities immediately set about a process of keeping the fulfilment of the agreement in indefinite pendency. In the words of Awadhesh, "then one has to organise another series of agitational activities to persue the agreement." At some stage in this process the project officers also start making individual overtures to the most vocal and inconvenient leaders and try to buy them off by offering inducements. To use Awadesh's idiom, "It then becomes very difficult for some of us to preserve our *Satitva*" (virtue). Another aspect of PAP agitations is that unlike labour unrest the State authorities either keep away from it or intervene merely from a law and order angle. This is directly traceable to the absence of a legal or policy base or responsibility for ensuring rehabilitation. This outline of agitations in the Bijpur area shows that inspite of efforts and negotiations with the project authorities the PAPs had to take recourse to public interest litigation in the Supreme Court to achieve some concrete results, even when the then Commissioner for Scheduled Castes and Scheduled Tribes, had visited the area and frankly criticised the projects' attitude.

The role of the elected representatives of the area in the State Assembly and the Parliament would also be germane to this discussion on leadership and agitations. The Parliamentary seat of this area is reserved for the Scheduled Castes. The sitting M.P. for most of the time when displacements took place was a person belonging to the Panika caste. Some of the informants freely expressed the view that he spoke, as if in two voices. He would usually support all the demands of the oustees in a village or general meeting, particularly in informal meetings with villagers. But often changed his stance consequently when he faced the project and other authorities. It was said that the M.P. even though thoroughly familiar with the people and the area never forcefully placed before the government and project authorities the real problem of the PAP—that these people should have been provided with *some land* at least to pursue the only vocation known to them. Had he pressed for it, lands could be identified for allocation to the oustees. A Gond, who has represented the reserved Assembly seat twice, emphasised that the area still had patches of land which could be developed by the government for the oustees. A clear impression was also gathered that all the project big-wigs, specially from the NTPC kept the M.P. happy through all the means at their disposal to ensure that he would keep the people 'under control' and dissuade them from impeding the project work.

8

THE LEGAL FRAME

AFTER having a fairly extensive picture of the empirical reality with regard to displacement and rehabilitation, it is pertinent to go through the legal frame. In this chapter, the various laws regarding land acquisition and forests would be analysed from both the projects' perspective and oustees' perspective. In Sonbhadra district the land obtained by the State Government (dam, reservoir), State enterprise (UPSEB), central corporations (NTPC, NCL) and companies (HINDALCO, Kanoria and the HiTech Carbon) is either forest land or revenue land under cultivation or forests, grazing land, *banjar*, etc. with the village panchayats, acquired under the Land Acuisition Act, 1894 and the Coal Bearing Areas (Acquisition and Development) Act, 1957.

The Land Acquisition Act 1894

The Land Acquisition Act, 1894 (LAA 1894) is a very old central law but it has remained in operation for a whole century with few amendments. The latest amendments were made by the Parliament in 1984 and some amendments have been made by the State legislatures from time to time.

We may briefly recapitulate here the salient provisions of this law. The Act aims to provide the law for the acquisition of land needed for public purposes. Section 3 relating to definitions does not comprehensively define the expression 'public purposes'. The 1984 amendment, however, lays down that, public purposes include provision of village site, land for town and rural planning, planned development of land from public funds, land to corporations controlled by the state, land for residential purposes to the poor or landless or to persons displaced or affected by any scheme undertaken by government/ corporation/local authority, land for building public office, etc. Government of U.P. added another clause in 1954 that public purpose includes the settlement of land for agriculture with weaker section of the people.

The procedure prescribed for acquisition of land and determination of compensation therefore is briefly :

(a) The Collector shall notify the specification of land likely to be needed for any public purpose or for a company. This notification shall be published in official gazette and two daily newspapers circulating in that locality, atleast one shall be in regional language and . . . public notice of the substance of the notification to be given at convenient places in the said locality. After this notification has been made, survey of land in question can be made by officers so authorised (Section 4).

(b) Objections to the proposed acquisition can be made within thirty days by any person interested in any land so notified (Section 5A). Government of U.P. have curtailed this period to twenty-one days through an amendment.

(c) Thereafter a declaration to the effect that land is acquired for public purposes shall be made (Section 6).

(d) Following this declaration the Collector shall be directed by the government to take orders for acquisition of land. The Collector shall

thereupon get the land marked out (Sections 7 and 8).

(e) This will be followed by the Collector's public notice to be given at convenient places and/or near the land and also to be served in writing to occupiers, etc. saying that the government intends to take possession of the land and that claims to compensation by all persons interested in such land may be made to him (Section 9).

(f) "Persons interested" include all persons claiming an interest in compensation to be made" . . . and "those interested in easement affecting the land" (Section 38). They also include "co-proprietor, sub-proprietor, mortgagee, tenant or otherwise" (Section 10).

(g) This will be followed by the enquiry into the objections by the persons having interest in the land and making an award of compensation by Collector (Section 11).

(h) The 1984 amendments provide that the award should be made within a period of two years from the date of public declaration and if this is not done the entire proceedings for the acquisition shall lapse. Government of U.P. have provided for correction of award by Collector within six months (Section 11A).

(i) In cases of urgency, whenever the appropriate government so directs, Collector can take possession of the land after expiry of fifteen days from the publication of the notice, even though no such awards have been made, after paying 80 per cent of his estimate of compensation (Section 17).

(j) The determination of compensation by Collector shall take into consideration the market value on the date of publication of the notice, damages due to taking any standing crops or trees, damages due to severing such land from the proprietor's other land, damages in respect of injurious effect to his other *property movable or immovable or his earnings,* and reasonable expenses incidental to change of residence or place of business (Section 23).

The Coal Bearing Areas (Acquisition and Development) Act, 1957

The NCL has its coalfields stretching from Audi onwards to the areas beyond Singrauli in M.P. In this area wherever coal is to be mined, land has to be acquired under the Coal Bearing Areas (Acquisition and Development) Act, 1957 (CBAA). The objective of this central law is 'to establish, in the economic interest of India, greater public control over the coal mines industry and its development.' It provides for the acquisition of "unworked land containing or likely to contain coal deposits or of rights in or over such land or for the extinguishment or modification" in the existing such rights.

The central government, under this law, appoints any person to be the Competent Authority (Section 3), for the purpose of this Act and, thereafter, the process of acquisition of any land or prospecting/mining rights in any land is pursued by this Competent Authority.

The process starts with a notification in the official gazette regarding the intention of acquiring the prospecting of coal in any land (Section 4). This notification extinguishes or modifies all prospecting licences (Section 5). Once the government is satisfied that coal is obtainable in the area notified under Section 4, a notification in the official gazette regarding its intention to acquire the area has to be given within two years from the date of the earlier notification (Section 7). Objections to this notification can be made within thirty days (Section 8). After considering the objections, etc. the government has to make a declaration to the effect that the land has been acquired (Section 9) and thereafter the right in such land "vest absolutely in the central government free from all encumbrances" (Section 10). These rights can also be vested by the government in a government company (Section 11). The other provisions for land acquisition, viz., compulsion, cash compensation only, persons entitled to compensation, etc. in the CBAA are the same as in the LAA.

As regards determination of compensation the CBAA provides that it can be fixed 'by agreement' or by a tribunal, consisting of a person who is or has been or is qualified to be a judge of High Court, constituted by the Central Government (Section 14). A Competent Authority presently functions in the NCL and a part time tribunal functions in the Civil Court, Mirzpur.

The Laws and Conditions in Sonbhadra

In the previous chapters, we have described the socio-economic conditions of the population affected by the land acquisitions made in the past thirty-five years. The entire district of Mirzapur was quite backward, remote and isolated by way of levels of agricultural income, communi-cation and other infrastructural facilities. It had remained so as it was a Partially Excluded Area during the colonical regime. Low levels of literacy, a mixed ethnic composition and traditional or tribal way of life are still the main characteristics of the people of southern Mirzapur, now Sonbhadra, thus leading to a 'fringe existence' (Majumdar 1960). To this may be added the fact that Mirzapur town (the district headquarters) was at a distance of more than 200 kilometres from the main theatres of industrialisation.

In this scenario the various steps of the acquisition procedure, such as public notifications in two newspapers and filing of objections, questioning 'public purpose' within twenty-one days, and declaration under Section 6 and notice to persons under Section 9 of the LAA, 1894 seem to assume rather hypothetical dimensions. Do the common tribals or Scheduled Caste persons residing in a remote village in the former Singrauli state really have the wherewithal to enter the arena against the mighty state? Can they ever challenge a declaration of 'public purpose' and properly place the grounds for the infirmity of such a declaration or suitably bring up the factors determining the compensation before the prescribed authority? In the areas where the NCL is interested, the land of the same person may fall under the provisions of CBAA for coal mining and under the LAA for being required for any other purpose. In such cases the person has to deal with two sets of authorities.

The data gathered through our family surveys and oustee profiles amply document this situation. Our informants had, however, found the CBAA machinery more responsive and their compensations better. A worker in the area stated that the Central Government had issued several notifications under the CBAA in 1957, 1965 and in 1974 but no information about them ever reached the residents of the area through handbills or beating of drums (*dondi*) and the period allowed for objections expired. Further, the land was valued for compensation with reference to the date of notification while prices went up mainfold, subsequently by the time compesation was actually paid. The near absence of sales of land in the Sonbhadra area before acquisition also created difficulties in determining valuation. It was therefore worked out by the collector and was on the low side, due to the quality of lands. In Jhingurda and Jayant Coal Mines of the NCL the payments of compensation remained pending due to the land owners objecting to the rate of valuation (Setu 1985). But, by and large, the NTPC and NCL paid higher compensations in the Sidhi district of M.P. as compared to Sonbhadra.

The very bases of the LAA 1984, its legal premises, its apparent incompatability with our constitutional frame of

Fundamental Rights, Directive Principles of State Policy and Special provisions for the Scheduled Castes/Tribes and weaker sections has been widely questioned. Further, LAA's failure to provide any compensation excepting cash and its not being applicable to a large category of weaker people in the rural polity who obtain their livelihood from the land but who are not recognised as having any 'interest' in that land under the LAA 1894 has also been strongly criticised by Commissioner (1990), Joshi (1987), Verma (1985), Fernandes and Thukral (1989), Singh (1989), Morse (1992), Roy Burman (1992), Dhagamwar (1989), Mahapatra (1991), and Baboo (1993) among many others.

Commissioner (1990) is of the view that during the British period when the state started establishing its authority over the natural resources, the authority of the community prevalent till then was extinguished. The tradition in our country to regard natural resources as 'means of livelihood and not property' was ignored and land was treated purely as property belonging to the individual. The LAA 1894 is largely based on 'the English Land Acquisition Act. But in U.K., unlike in India, the laws of compensation make liabilities fully justiciable in accordance with the actual value of the property to the individual' (Singh 1989).

What has happened after the independence was that anything and everything was given the name of development. Therefore, it has been possible to use LAA 1894 for almost all sorts of programmes including even tourist resorts for the affluent. EDF (1990) quotes the example of land acquisition for an "over sized airport" in Sonbhadra. Dhagamwar (1989) points out that the 1984 amendments to LAA 1894 have made land acquisitions much easier. Now the public sector can directly acquire land and the private sector can do so through the government. Earlier they had to purchase land at market prices. Lands can even be acquired for residential colonies. Under LAA 1894 the only entitlement for the persons whose land is acquired is cash compensation. The determination of compensation is also not equitable particularly in respect of tribal and backward areas where land is not freely sold. This is specially true of Sonbhadra because the entire south of Kaimur range was a Partially Excluded Area till the Constitution was adopted. Even after its becoming an ordinary area much of the titles to the land suffered from infirmities, which will be discussed later in this chapter. Therefore at the time of acquiring land for the Rihand Dam in 1960 the government decided to correlate compen-sation to the *lagan* (land revenue). Then, within a decade or so how the area became so 'normal' that market prices of land could determine a fair compensation? Can it be expected that land transactions were taking place at the time of notification regarding acquisition, in a free and fair manner. The substantial difference between the rates of compensations paid by the NCL and the NTPC for acquisitions in the same vicinity also indicate that the yardsticks adopted were rather arbitrary. Large tract of land was also presumed to be forest land and as per LAA 1894 cultivators of forest land along with landless labourers, artisans etc. are not regarded as persons interested (MARG 1990). "In the opinion of independent lawyer the prices paid for land is about half of its market value" (EDF 1990).

"Therefore, when in pursuance of these incongruous principles and in a depressed psychological frame, the entire land of a farmer which is 'life personified for him', so much so that he is prepared to die or kill even when a field-boundary is disturbed by someone, is snatched away under the shadow of the authority of the state, merely by throwing at him some rupee coins, numbering a hundred or two, he is hurt to the core, but cannot express his anguish. In a state of utter helplessness; he may get deeply disturbed and prefer to end his life. But the powers that be do not see in this even a shadow of injustice anywhere around them, everything appears to be proper and equitable, when looked at with spectacles of formal justice and the transaction may even be considered to be in his interest" (Commissioner 1990). "We heard some strange comments from the officers responsible for assessing the property" . . . such as "that's quite good enough for yokels like you", "it's very good of the government to pay you anything", "you don't deserve as much", and particularly to low-caste people, "why do you have such fine houses (or permanent homes)—do you need such things?" (EDF 1990). One wonders as to what this law is about and for whom does this system stand ?

Singh (1989) argues that land laws in India, in violation Article 14 of the Constitution—equality before the law—have generated two types of citizens. The first type are having right to land as they are governed by the tenancy laws and the second category is of those who do not get any title of land however long they may live on it or cultivate it as they are governed by the forest laws. Further, the forest laws infringe on another basic right of the forest-dwellers, viz. right to life enshrined in Article 21. This dispensation discriminates the most against the tribals. Singh also refers to the Human Right Convention, International Labour Convention 107 and Convention of Aboriginal Rights to all of which India is a signatory.

The right of the oustees to fair compensation for their loss of livelihood and the onus on the state to provide effective rehabilitation measures are also relatable to the extended interpretation of Article 21, 39(2) and (f), 41 and 42 of the Constitution. A Constitution Bench of the Supreme Court has held that the right to life includes the right to livelihood, that is the means of livelihood. The Court reasoned that, 'if the right to livelihood is not treated as a part of the constitutional right to life, the easiest way of depriving a person of his right to life would be to deprive him of his means of livelihood to the point of abrogation' (Sorabjee 1995). It also includes, inter alia, right to educational facilities, conditions of freedom and dignity and humane conditions of work, as also the right to free legal aid to poor or indigent persons also in the vital context of PAPs.

The tribals are, in many areas, regarded as encroachers on forest lands and the government from time to time agrees as a kind of benevolent act to regularise their occupancy and the Narmada Tribunal Award underwriting the intention of the Government of Gujarat to do so is a case in point. In Sonbhadra however, the legal position has undergone a change due to two decisions of the Supreme Court—the first relating to survey and settlement operations taking into account the *rights* of the tribal cultivators in forest lands and the other judgement awarding interim cash compensation to the cultivators of such lands by the NTPC.

As Baxi (1989) points out, our Constitution "celebrates the Spirit of *Swaraj* meaning participatory governance" . . . It is a Republican India where Indian citizen stands endowed with rights and responsibilities for the development of the country. By 'development' the Constitution means simply that process of governance which, while respecting human rights of all persons, secures to all Indians freedom from material impoverishment. The planning process in India however, betrays the spirit of the Indian Constitution . . . and In no area is this 'singular' inversion of the Constitution more acutely demonstrated than, perhaps, in the decisions concerning large, medium and small irrigation projects".

Discussing the implementation of the process of land acquisition under LAA 1894, Commissioner (1990) brings out how the objections of the people to the validity of 'public purpose' in respect of land to be acquired are disposed of by the authorities in a routine way. Moreover, the objections under this provision cannot be raised by the people in general or the community but only by those who have interest in the land and how the definition of interest in the land (sections 10 and 38, LAA 1894) is quite narrow has been discussed earlier in this section. Our sample of oustees brought out many cases of people not even being served notices regarding the acquisition of their lands.

The displacements in the tribal areas throw up the question discussed above in a particularly acute manner. These areas are characterised, *inter alia*, by being "outside the market system" . . .; dependence on forests or in other words living in "semi isolation . . ." and "independent of national economic system. . ."; "their economic life style largely dependent on the specific natural environment; . . . and having loose tenure over their traditional lands . . ." (Morse 1992).

Problem of Land and Tribal Unrest

The foregoing discussions relating to certain legal aspects of the land *vis-a-vis* the cultivators specially the tribals and Scheduled Castes in Sonbhadra district calls for a full exposition of facts in a historical perspective.

In the south of Kaimur, the tribal area of the district, there are 433 villages, 134 in Robertsganj Tahsil and 299 in Dudhi Tehsil. Like extensive tribal areas in other parts of India (India 1986), survey and settlement operations had not been updated or properly completed in these areas. Whatever records existed were prepared on the basis of *Nazri Paimaish* (visual estimate of boundaries). The main reasons for the situation were the inaccessibility of the area, the practice of shifting cultivation, and customary granting of the rights of cultivation to the tillers by the *Supurdar* (in Dudhi Government State) and zamindars in the feudatory states. Thus there were thousands of cultivators, generally tribals, who had been cultivating their agricultural plot for more than a century without any proper record of rights. Under the circumstances, the extension of U.P. Zamindari Abolition and Lands Reforms Act, 1950 to Sonbhadra conferring the proprietory rights on the tillers also failed to provide any relief to them.

Thus, while many of the tribal cultivators had some kind of 'loose tenure' over the land through entries in the far from complete land records as 'cultivators without any title', the government decided to transfer the entire area deemed to be *banjar* or forest to the Forest Department. Notifications under Section 4 of the Indian Forest Act, 1927 (IFA) were issued in respect of 7.89 lakh acres of land, out of a total area of 13.72 lakh acres. Further, nearly one lakh acre were notified under Section 20 of the Indian Forest Act, 1927 as reserved forests. While these develop-ments were going on, industrialisation began and the government began allotting land deemed to be under the Forest Department to various industrial units, including the private ones. Then, the oustees of Rihand dam which submerged 106 villages (1.06 lakh acre) were also asked by the authorities to occupy the land managed by the Forest Department in the neighbourhood of the submerged villages, without being given any *patta* or preparing a record of demarcation. Moreover, the government also donated one lakh acres of land in the same area for Bhoodan purposes. All these decisions created a chaotic situation where traditional tillers, Rihand oustees, allottees of Bhoodan land, etc. started claiming the same patches of land. Since considerable denudation of forests had taken place in the meantime and industrialisation had brought in migrants in large number, grabbing of tribal lands became rampant on a large scale.

The National Agricultural Commission visited the area and stressed in its report of February 1972 the urgent need for expeditious settlement of the problem. But during 70s the government, instead of taking up survey and preparation of records of rights on an urgent basis, set up committees to examine the question and simply issued orders for taking up survey and settlement operations without actually ensuring an implementation in the field.

In 1981 Indian the Forest Act was amended under which the Government of India assumed all powers to denotify areas under reserved forest and diversion of forest areas to non-forest purposes, taking away the state government's authority to do so. As a result of this move the Forest Department started applying the law stringently and thousands of cases were initiated in Sonbhadra against tillers of the land who had been there for generations. This was the beginning of unrest among the tribals and led to the Banwasi Sewa Ashram conducting a sample survey in five villages to identify cases of undeserved eviction by the forest officers. Thereafter they filed a public interest litigation in the Supreme Court in July 1982 and the Supreme Court issued an interim order laying down a time schedule of about three months for completing the survey operations and banning all evictions of Adivasi, Harijans and Backward Caste cultivators. The Supreme Court also said that a high power body should be appointed to settle various disputes on the spot to protect customary rights of the tribals and other farmers.

The State Government sought time from the apex court regarding the survey operations and appointed a high level committee to examine the status of land records in the area (Maheswar Prasad Committee). The Committee submitted its report in December 1983. It confirmed the state of "dissatisfaction in the minds of the people" and felt that "it may lead to serious problem of law and order". They also delared the notifications declaring reserved forest being "without jurisdiction" Further, they recommended the immediate creation of a Special Agency to undertake survey and record operations. This Agency should not only accept all the entries made in the incomplete land record operations of 1964-65 under

'Varg-4' (cultivation of forest lands) as proof of occupancy but also recommended acceptance of occupancies in the field as seen during the survey to be treated as sufficient for settlement of such lands with the tillers, within the limits prescribed by the land ceiling law. The Committee stated that out of a total area of 13.93 lakh acres in the 1422 villages of the two tahsils of Sonbhadra district 9.23 lakh acres lay south of Kaimur. Of this 7.89 lakh acres had been notified under Section 4 IFA and 0.99 lakh acres thereof were notified as Reserved Forest as well. Only 0.45 lakh acres of this was entered under *Varg-4* in revenue records. During a spot verification the Committee found that 27,705 persons were found cultivating the land. Of them 53 per cent were Scheduled Castes and Adivasis. No record operations had been undertaken in 177 villages (1.72 lakh acres) till 1983 (U.P. 1983).

After the submission of the Maheswar Prasad Committee report in December 1983, once again the Government of U.P. delayed acting upon it. A delegation waited upon the Chief Minister to plead for early action without any result. This led to a widespread agitation by the tribals leading to the formation of a *Morcha*. A peaceful *Rasta Roko* was organised which was violently dealt with by the administration. The situation drew extensive adverse comments for the government from the media and activists.

The Banwasi Sewa Ashram petitioned the Supreme Court for orders, drawing their attention to the prevailing situation in the area. The Supreme Court then issued an order which :

- *(i)* provides for a record and settlement operations to be conducted;
- *(ii)* sets a time frame for completing the processes;
- *(iii)* envisages complete forest land settlement and opportunities to every one to file claims;
- *(iv)* appoints a Board of Commissioners to supervise

record and settlement operations and oversee the implementation of the direction given by the Court;

(v) appoints the petitioner himself (Prembhai) as one of the Commissioners, thus accepting his third party status and his commitment and competence to protect the legal rights of Adivasis;

(vi) asks the State Government to appoint five experienced Additional District Judges and an adequate number of record officials;

(vii) stipulates that procedural and legal aid should be made available to all claimants at the cost of the State Government, and directs the State Government to deposit a sum of Rs. 5 lakhs with the District Legal Aid Committee headed by the District Judge of Mirzapur; and

(viii) permits the District Legal Aid Committee to provide legal aid either by itself or through any Social Action Group like the Banwasi Seva Ashram.

The Government of U.P. have since appointed a staff of more than 800 persons for the survey and land record operations which are still going on. In the meantime the Supreme Court have also ordered in November 1986 that the Bijpur Unit of NTPC should pay interim compensation at agreed rates to persons recorded as cultivating forest land *(Varg-4)* as per the 1964-65 records (Varma and Prembhai 1987) and subsequently made the order final in February 1992. However, this interim compensation had not been received by the PAPs till the time of our study.

9

SEARCH FOR A POLICY

DEVELOPING countries have embarked upon a variety of large projects for the purpose of expanding and extending irrigation, power generation, industries and infrastructural facilities such as highways, airports, railways, etc. "India is currently the developing country with the largest dam construction programme and correspondingly with the most massive involuntary displacement . . ." (Cernea 1990). What Cernea has postulated here is only the displacement and rehabilitation aspects of the projects. Some other allied issues would be, ensuring that the large projects—mining, irrigation, industrial, power generation, etc.—should be formulated and implemented so as to ensure that they prove to be people friendly, environment friendly and actively endeavour to promote the interests of the tribal oustees as well as their hinterland. Right from the stage of formulation they should have in-built systems which will be responsive to people's needs and actively advance their interest along with macro development. They should not under any circumstances create or aggravate inequalities in the tribal areas and disbalance the eco-systems. If such an approach is not followed, these could be aptly labelled as "the 'internal' colonialism of India (relative to the tribals') . . ." (Mendelsohn and Baxi 1994).

Even though the counter-developmental consequences of population displacement bringing about impoverishment in all its varied dimensions has now become well-known through "independent sociological, anthropological, and environmental investigation on resettlement" (Cernia 1990) there are very few governments who "have pursued an appropriate national policy setting the basic norms to be observed in forced population displacement. I am aware of such formally adopted policies only in Indonesia, Turkey and China. That the number is so limited represents in itself an indication of pervasive underestimation and absence of policy response by the State" (*Ibid.*, 1990).

The absence of a national policy frame in India has been commented upon strongly in almost all the studies on the subject (Commissioner 1990; Morse 1992; Fernandes and Thukral 1989; Fernandes and Raj 1992; Joshi 1987) and others. The unusual delay in finalising a national policy after repeatedly announcing that a policy was on the anvil seems to convey a message that the government is reluctant to adopt a comprehensive national policy. Cernea (1991) aptly points out, "Some of the State governments have adopted policy frameworks but a national policy for the entire country is long over due".

The failure to prepare any national policy brings us to a position where various local authorities, ministries, departments and public sector corporations, who get land acquired for their projects as a 'public purpose', through land acquisition law come to adopt a variety of approaches and measures for the settlement of PAPs. We have discussed earlier that the Sonbhadra scenario of industrialisation; dam construction for irrigation, and power projects involves, almost all types of agencies. Therefore, it is essential to briefly discuss the different guidelines, instructions, adopted policies or statements from the agencies concerned in this regard. These can be of general application to all PAPs, irrespective of their status as Scheduled Castes/Tribes, etc. or particularly focusing on the Scheduled Castes/Tribes due to their constitutional status or both.

Government of India

Ministry of Water Resources

In May 1986, the Ministry of Energy and Irrigation (Department of Irrigation) issued guidelines for the rehabilitation of persons displaced due to major reservoir projects. These guidelines referred to the Prime Minister's 'wish that the displaced persons' interest should be created in the project itself by assigning them government and other waste lands in the command area. Where such lands were not available it would be worthwhile to think of a system, atleast the larger landholders in the command area are *compelled* to part with some land for this purpose. Such a step would need legislative backing on the lines of Maharashtra. The Maharashtra Resettlement of Project Displaced Persons Act 1976, *inter alia* incorporates some commendable features : a comprehensive definition of project; a liberal definition of 'displaced person' to include agricultural labourer; creation of a Directorate of Resettlement with powers to ensure speedy resettlement; as far as possible land to be given to displaced persons, and a better formula for determining compensation. The States, were requested to keep this directive in view so as to ensure protection of the weakest sections specially the tribals.

Ministry of Home Affairs

The Ministry of Home Affairs was earlier the nodal ministry for safeguarding the interests of the Scheduled Castes/Tribes. Even though the report of the Scheduled Areas and Scheduled Tribes Commission (1961) and several annual reports of the Commissioner for Scheduled Castes and Scheduled Tribes had made many significant recommendations for guarding the displaced persons, particularly the Scheduled Tribes from discomfort and anxiety, the Ministry took a long time in formulating a set of guidelines. The guidelines first issued in the year 1982 stated that "in the past adequate care had hardly been taken to plan a satisfactory rehabilitation of tribals displaced from their ancestral land" and went on to lay down that for the successful rehabilitation of displaced tribals adoption of the following measures may *be considered* :

- *(i)* The compensation needs to be determined on the basis of a new formula because tribal lands are not sold in free transactions due to protective laws. The tribals should not be evicted without full payment of compensation and they should also be helped in purchasing alternative land. Excessive acquisition of land should not be done and emergency measures should not be taken for acquisition.
- *(ii)* The tribal families should be provided with alternative land, atleast to some extent and they should not be uprooted from their traditional occupations.
- *(iii)* Project report for settlement of local communities should be prepared well in advance by personnel conversant with their cultural traditions and they should be rehabilitated as a community.
- *(iv)* If land is not provided, employment should be provided to atleast one person in each family for which a substantial training programme should be undertaken while the participants are already taken on muster rolls of the project.
- *(v)* Free, developed house-sites, primary school buildings, community centres, medical care and drinking water must be provided.
- *(vi)* Training programme for entrepreneurial skills,

with follow-up by way of ensuring financial support, marketing outlets, supply of raw material, etc. should be built up to develop alternative occupations.

(vii) A law similar to Maharashtra may be enacted by other States.

Bureau of Public Enterprises (BPE)

In February 1986, the Bureau of Public Enterprises which oversees the working of the public sector undertakings of the Government of India issued guidelines in order to bring about uniformity of approach in regard to acquisition of land and other related aspects of projects, in the public sector, departmental as well as those directly executed by the Central Government. The salient features of these guidelines were :

(i) Effort should be made to avoid acquisition of valuable agricultural land, forest land or ecologically fragile land so as to minimise disturbance to human habitations. The quantum of acquisition should be minimum and further expansion should not be allowed to increase this minimum by more than 25 per cent.

(ii) The administrative ministries/departments should undertake a survey to identify surplus lands acquired by the undertakings under them. The land thus identified should be transferred for new public sector undertakings and associated activities.

(iii) Expert agencies should be consulted in order to minimise fresh acquisition of land and efforts made to provide common services, etc. In the contiguously located undertakings.

(iv) The procedure for payment of compensation should be streamlined, its level raised to the 1984 amendments to the Land Acquisition Act,

1894; and it should be paid within a reasonable time.

(v) Each land acquisition unit should have a small rehabilitation cell. The cost of this cell should be borne by the project.

(vi) The project authorities should examine the list of displaced families received from the rehabilitation cell with reference to their educational attainments and arrange for imparting education and training in existing institutions at the cost of the project or in special institutions to equip them for being considered for employment. The training will not, however, be a commitment for ultimate employment.

(vii) Rehabilitation cells will monitor the progress of rehabilitation and in case of tribals and Scheduled Castes Ministry of Welfare and Ministry of Environment and Forest would also be associated with the preparation of rehabilitation scheme.

The above guidelines, *significantly*, also lay down that any understanding, informal or formal to provide employment to one person in each displaced family will stand withdrawn. But project authorities may help the state governments in creating avenues for avocations like poultry farming for the oustees. Guideline (ii) clearly reveals that many projects have been acquiring lands much in excess of their needs. But it does not allow such excess lands being used for relief to the oustees.

The guidelines summarised above, all seem to address a post-project situation and none has gone comprehensively into the question of how industrialisation, through heavy industries, mining projects and even thermal projects, in the tribal areas can be so tailored as to benefit the displaced tribal people as well as the affected tribal hinterlands. But B.D. Sharma had given thought to the need for such an approach prior to these guidelines when the strategy of Tribal Sub Plan (TSP) was shaped. He spelt out a comprehensive approach (Sharma 1975) which has basic strength to ensure that industrial development benefits both the PAPs and the tribal hinterlands. His plan starts right from a stage when any industrial activity of a sizeable nature is planned for a tribal area. In other words planning for the benefit of the tribals should, according to him, begin from the stage of project formulation for the industry itself or even from the very time that its idea is floated. The strategy evolves through various stages like preparing the tribal community for the proposed industrialisation, both psychologically and materially, through carefully planned measures to build up a 'skill-spectrum' of the tribals after due identification and advance education and training process accordingly. Further, it also envisages entrepreneurship building among carefully selected young educated groups in the tribal community. This section would be developed through a supportive institutional frame of co-operatives and individual enterprises achieved with help from the banks, small industries service agencies, etc., to derive maximum benefit from self employment avenues likely to be created in the process of industrialisation. Then, he has also spelt out how small business like contract work, eateries, canteens, tea shops, etc. can be taken up by even untrained tribals right from the initial stages of transition in the area. Further on in time, small ancillary units and other such activities can be set up by the tribals themselves as a part of the industrial complex. As regards the hinterlands, he speaks of adaptative linkages with local economy so that these areas benefit from demands for vegetables, dairy products, poultry, etc. In conclusion, he emphasises the need for the personnel in the industry to appreciate the distinctive socio-economic environment around them and also their understanding of the tribal world view specially in the realm of staticism versus modern mobility in order to avoid any mismatch of the two worlds extensively seen in the project affected tribal areas. Unfortunately none of the central ministries/ agencies show any trace of this strategy.

Government of Uttar Pradesh

The policy frame for rehabilitation of the Government of Uttar Pradesh has undergone changes from time to time. The first project was the construction of Rihand Dam started in 1947-48. It appears from the reports connected with the area that till then the Government of U.P. had not adopted any policy for rehabilitation of displaced persons. Since the land to be acquired was unsurveyed and carried hereditary rates of land revenue, it was decided in November 1956 that special rates of cash compensation for land in the area should be fixed for the various categories of cultivators of the lands. These were one hundred times the land revenue for *Bhumidars*, thirty times for *Sirdars* and five to nine times the land revenue for the *Adhivasis* and *Asamis*.

In December 1973, the Government of U.P., taking into consideration the difficulties faced by the oustees whose lands are acquired, ordered that :

(i) Immediate arrangement should be made for the rehabilitation of people whose lands are acquired, and atleast one person each from such families should be provided employment.

(ii) Those whose residential premises are acquired should be provided with houses to be built by the department which acquires the house.

(iii) The expenditure on the construction of the house should be included in the project cost and employment should also be provided in the same project as far as possible.

(iv) The extent of land to be acquired for any

project should be minimum possible and *usar* and *banjar* land should be used for the purpose as far as possible.

(*v*) The project buildings and staff quarters should be more than one storey high so that the quantum of land required is reduced.

The Collectors and all government departments including the undertakings under them were asked to ensure that the oustee families were assured rehabilitation on the above lines without any delay. In February 1980, it was further decided that the 'at least one' job to be provided to oustee families by the project responsible for the displacement should be according to qualification, without any restriction on the pay scale and in January 1981, 'family' was defined to include besides the displaced person, his/her wife/husband, unmarried sons/daughters, married sons, grandsons, unmarried grand-daughters and dependent father/mother.

However, the instructions issued by different departments are at variance with the State Government's rehabilitation approach. The Irrigation Department is constructing the Kanhar Dam in Sonbhadra and the Tehri Dam in Tehri-Garhwal district. While for the Kanhar Dam oustees nothing except cash compensation is being provided, the Tehri Dam project estimate itself includes attractive 'rehabilitation packages' for the Tehri town oustees and the rural people as an integral part of the project. For the rural people it includes not less than two acres developed land for the acquired land and also for the landless, cash compensation as assessed or ex-gratia payment @ Rs. 12,000 per acre for irrigated and Rs. 4,000 per acre for unirrigated lands, compensation and ex-gratia payment for buildings, displacement grant, supply of building material at stock-issue rates and rehabilitation grant to restart agricultural operations.

Besides, the families will move as communities and the new villages to be established will have all necessary amenities like roads, schools, community centres, dispensaries, stockmen centres and electricity (Hasan 1985). This example amply shows how a set of instructions issued by the State Government have been totally ignored in a tribal area by its own department and followed gene-rously in a non-tribal area by the same department. Obviously the Tehri Dam PAPs got such a deal because they have been vocal and agitative while the tribals of Sonbhadra received a raw deal because they are backward, ignorant and lack a dynamic leadership.

Corporations

Northern Coalfields Limited (Central Coalfields Limited)

Northern Coalfields Limited, replying to our question whether they had adopted any policy relating to effective rehabilitation of displaced persons stated as below :

> As per guidelines of Government of India issued in 1984-85 suitable house site in size between 0.01 ha. to 0.02 ha. is being provided to those whose houses are required to be shifted. However, in NCL a plot of 60′ x 40′ (0.024 ha.) is provided to each family who are required to be shifted.
> Preference in employment is given to the land oustees depending upon the requirement of the Projects. So far, NCL has been able to offer employment to the project affected persons with landholding as low as :
> For general Classes — 0.50 acres or more
> For S.C./S.T. — 0.02 acres or more".

National Thermal Power Corporation (NTPC)

The National Thermal Power Project is a gigantic public

sector undertaking with power projects working or in the process of being set up in different parts of the country. In reply to our question whether they had adopted any policy relating to effective rehabilitation of displaced persons, the Singrauli Super Thermal Power Plant, Shaktinagar gave a rather ambiguous reply simply stating that, 'they had a policy for rehabilitating the PAPs'. They, in a personal discussion, indicated that actually a policy had been drawn up but not adopted formally by the Board of Directors. But the power stations had been told by the corporate office to act in accordance with that policy. However, the policy was a recent one and the Singrauli power station was found to be still in a stage of planning to implement it.

Suprisingly, the management of the Rihand Thermal Power Station, Bijpur, the second NTPC power house in the area studied were reluctant to give us any information whatsoever in the matter. They wrote that all the information in this regard was to be had only from the state authorities concerned. However, their Deputy General Manager, in the course of a brief talk claimed in a sweeping statement that "the people here were uncivilized . . . had not seen even a motor truck before we came to this area . . . and we have provided them with all facilities like plots, drinking water, electric light and job".

In May 1993, the NTPC announced its rehabilitation and resettlement policy. The preamble of this policy states (NTPC 1993) that since most of the NTPC Projects are located in remote areas, NTPC will take measures to resettle and rehabilitate Project Affected Persons (PAPs) with the objective that they will improve or at least regain their previous PP standard of living. As and when any National Rehabilitation and Resettlement (R&R) guidelines/policy/government order is finalized and adopted, NTPC will review and modify its R&R policy.

The policy statement, *inter alia*, admits that "improper resettlement and rehabilitation is the root of discontentment and alienation of the PAPs" and "It may be difficult to operate a project efficiently without the cooperation of the local people". The action plan incorporates the goal of PAPs regaining their economic base and improve or at least regain their previous standard of living, earning capacity and production levels. The transition gap is to be reduced to a minimum.

This policy is divided into two parts. The first part is action plan designed for the future projects of the NTPC. This plan takes special care of the tribals simply by saying that 'Tribals will receive attention to restore their income'. Since the NTPC projects in Sonbhadra do not fall in this category, the second part of policy that deals with "earlier NTPC projects" only is of direct relevance, which states :

(i) One of the Corporate Objectives of the NTPC is social responsibility in respect of environmental protection and rehabilitation. Even earlier, NTPC has been making a conscious effort to rehabilitate the oustees by providing them with regular employment with NTPC, jobs with contractors, allotment of shops, award of petty contracts, etc. in a limited measure, apart from physically resettling the homestead of the oustees by allotting them developed plots of land. However, NTPC is strengthening the Community Development facilities to benefit the people living around its project area.

(ii) With respect to PAPs from earlier NTPC projects, NTPC will undertake special socio-economic surveys to ascertain the PAPs present socio-economic status. On the basis of these surveys and where found necessary, NTPC will, in consultation with said PAPs and appropriate State authorities, formulate a remedial action plan which would (a) focus on

developing or enhancing community facilities; (b) provide training and other facilities to upgrade skills and improve employment opportunities for PAPs; and (c) use its good offices to assist PAPs to achieve such improvements through ongoing government assistance programmes such as the Integrated Rural Development Programme.

(iii) In the locations/rehabilitation colonies where the conglomeration of PAPs exist community facilities, viz., primary school, dispensary, drinking water sells, link road connection to main road, village roads and area and road lighting would be provided.

(iv) One of the villages in the vicinity of the project area will be adopted to develop it as a model village.

The World Bank

Power projects of the NTPC are assisted by the World Bank and therefore the policy of the World Bank pertaining to the resettlement of displaced persons particularly tribals assumes relevance. It is also of great significance because the Bank has evolved it on the basis of an extremely wide range of sociological inputs of data and analysis, from tribal and other areas all over the world (Cernea 1990a and b, 1991, 1992; Morse 1992; Verma 1985). In February 1980, the World Bank issued its resettlement policy entitled 'Social Issues Associated with Involuntary Resettlement in Bank-Financed Projects'. Then, in October 1986 the Bank, after evaluating how the guidelines were being applied, issued a new Operational Policy Note, considerably strengthening the earlier policy. In 1988 the Bank first went public with the publication of its integrated and expanded policy-cum-technical paper.

This resettlement policy was again revised and issued

as an Operational Directive in June 1990 (World Bank 1990; Cernea 1991b). The main points of the policy are :

(i) Involuntary displacement should be avoided or minimized because of its disruptive and impoverishing effects. To avoid displacement, all viable alternative project designs should be explored. Where displacement is unavoidable, resettlement plans should be formulated with due care given to peoples' entitlements, needs and to environmental protection.

(ii) All involuntary resettlement should be conceived and executed as a development programme, providing sufficient opportunities to assist resettlers in their efforts to improve their former living standards and earning capacity, or at least to restore them. Displaced persons should be : (a) compensated for their losses at replacement cost, (b) given opportunities to share in project created benefits, and (c) assisted with the move and the transition period at the relocation site.

(iii) Allocation of adequate public sector resources (financial, technical, institutional) should be sufficient for compensating the losses incurred by those displaced and for ensuring the means for adequate resettlement and rehabilitation.

(iv) Displaced people should be assisted to move in groups, as social units of different kinds, so as to preserve as much as possible (and if desired by the affected people) the pre-existent social networks and local forms of organizations. Group or individual self-resettlement should be facilitated whenever it represents the preferred option.

(v) Minimizing the distance between the departure and the relocation sites can facilitate the

adaptation and integration of resettlers into the surrounding socio-cultural and natural environ-ments provided the economic and natural resource potential at the new site is adequate. However, the possibilities of tradeoffs between spatial/cultural distance and economic opportunities must be taken into account and balanced carefully.

(vi) The existing social and cultural institutions of resettlers and their hosts should be relied upon in conducting the displacement, transfer, and re-establishment process. Consultation and information to those to be displaced about their entitlements, options, moving schedules, etc. should be ensured throughout the preparation and relocation process. Community participation in planning and implementing resettlement should be encouraged and organized.

(vii) The new communities of the resettlers, often created by regrouping several prior smaller villages, should be designed as viable settlement systems equipped with infrastructure and services, with due consideration to their integration in the encompassing regional economic contexts.

(viii) Host communities that receive resettlers should be taken into account in the overall planning process and assisted to overcome possible adverse social and environmental consequences from increased population density.

(ix) Indigenous people, ethnic minorities, pastoralists, and other groups that may have informal customary rights to the land or other resources taken for the project must be provided with adequate land, infrastructure and other compensation. The absence of a formal legal title to land by such groups should not be

grounds for denying compensation and rehabilitation.

Tied to these policy provisions are procedural requirements. The most important of these is that the Bank cannot appraise and approve financing any major project that will cause the displacement unless it has received and reviewed a concrete resettlement plan that shows how the borrower will meet the policy objectives, how much it will cost, and when it will be completed.

Simultaneously, the World Bank also applied itself to framing a tribal component to supplement its general policy guidelines, as experience had shown that unless special measures were adopted, tribal people were more likely to be harmed than helped by development projects intended for beneficiaries other than themselves. An Operational Manual Statement dealing with tribal population was first issued in February 1982. The term "Tribal people" defined to cover ethnic groups typically with stable, low-energy, sustenance yield economic systems, as exemplified by hunter-gatherers, shifting or semipermanent farmers, herders, or fishermen who exhibit in varying degrees many of the characteristics, and the situation already discussed in Chapter 3.

Briefly, the Bank Policy is that :

(i) The Bank will assist projects only when satisfied that the borrower or relevant government agency supports and can implement measures that will effectively safeguard the integrity and well-being of the tribal people. Measures at either extreme—that perpetuate isolation from the national society and needed social services; or those promoting forced accelerated acculturation unsuited to the future well-being of the affected tribal people—should be avoided.

(ii) The programme for such projects will include

: (a) the recognition, demarcation and protection of tribal areas containing those resources required to sustain the tribal peoples' traditional means of livelihood; (b) appropriate social services that are in consonance with the tribe's acculturation status, including, especially, protection against diseases and the maintenance of health; (c) the maintenance to the extent desired by the tribe, of its cultural integrity and embodiments therefor; and (d) a forum for the participation of the tribal people in decisions affecting them, providing for adjudication and redress of grievances.

(iii) The design of an appropriate tribal component depends upon detailed, contemporary knowledge of the peoples to be affected. To the extent that project designers are unfamiliar with the affected tribal people pre-investment studies will be necessary, employing qualified indigenists and related disciplines.

It is presumed that the Bank's policies regarding resettlement form a conditionality to their assistance. The pressure exerted by the World Bank rather than the guidelines issued by the Government of India gradually produced some change for the better in the NTPC projects in Sonbhadra. Our study indicated that the approach to rehabilitation was somewhat better in the case of Bijpur power plant which came up in mid-80s, as compared to the Shaktinagar plant set up earlier. But as compared to say NCL, 'NTPC rehabilitation has been realised to be poor' (EDF 1990).

Supreme Court's Directives

Banwasi Seva Ashram, Govindpur has been in the forefront of the fight for the rights of the tribals, specially their land rights, in Sonbhadra district for the last two decades. This NGO has almost single-handedly created a movement among the tribals.

In 1982, the Ashram initiated a public interest case before the Supreme Court of India. Basically, it related to the complicated issue pertaining to the tribal lands. Since some of these lands had been acquired by the NTPC for its Bijpur plant and the Supreme Court ordered for a *status quo ante* (the NTPC had to get itself impleaded as a party in the writ petition and claimed that the completion of the project was a time bound programme and as such the land earmarked for the project be made free from prohibitive directions of the Court. Subsequently the Court disposed of the matter finally in February 1992. So far as the NTPC was concerned, the Court directed them to take the following measures to rehabilitate the evictees who were in actual physical possession of the lands, houses, etc. taken by the NTPC :

(i) One plot of land measuring 60′ × 40′ to each of the evictee families be distributed for housing purposes through the district administration.

(ii) Shifting allowance of Rs. 1500 and in addition a lumpsum grant of Rs. 3000 towards housing be given to each of the evictee families.

(iii) Free transportation be provided for shifting.

(iv) Monthly subsistence allowance equivalent to loss of net income from the acquired land to be determined by the District Judge, Sonbhadra subject to a maximum of Rs. 750 for a period of 10 years. The said payment shall not be linked with employment or any other compensation.

(v) Unskilled and semi-skilled posts in the project shall be reserved for the evictees subject to their eligibility and suitability.

(vi) The NTPC shall give preference to the oustees in employment in class III and IV posts under

its administration subject to their suitability and eligibility.

(vii) The evictees be offered employment through the contractors engaged by the NTPC.

(viii) The jobs of contractors under the administration of the NTPC be offered to the evictees.

(ix) The shops and other business premises within the NTPC campus be offered to the evictees.

(x) The NTPC shall operate for the benefit of the evictees self generating employment schemes such as carpentry training (free tools to be provided after completion of training), carpet weaving training, sericulture, masonry training, dairy farming, poultry farming and basket weaving training, etc.

(xi) The NTPC shall provide in the rehabilitation areas facilities such as *pucca* roads, *pucca* drainage system, hand pumps, wells, potable water supply, primary school, health centre, *panchayat bhavan,* electricity connections, bank and Sulabh Shauchalaya complex, etc.

(xii) The NTPC shall also provide hospitals, schools, adult education classes and sports centres for the evictees.

Further, the Supreme Court fixed the provisional land compensation @ Rs. 10,000 per acre and Rs. 850 per acre per year for the crops. They also directed that the District Judge, Sonbhadra shall be the authority to determine the claims for compensation in respect of land, crop, house and any other legitimate claims based on existing rights of the oustees. The District Judge, Sonbhadra was also to decide finally the list of evictees after scrutinising the lists submitted by the NTPC and verification in the field by the Commissioner appointed by the Supreme Court. The Court directed that the 'finally determinative' verification be completed expeditiously by 'probably March 1993'.

National Policy Goal (NPG)

The preceding discussion has amply brought out the fact that though guidelines are numerous and the directions multipronged, there has been no uniformity in either the policy or the implementation of the guidelines. Moreover, the much sought after goal of a national policy is still elusive. The Report of the Working Group on Development and Welfare of Scheduled Tribes during Eighth Five Year Plan (India 1989) discussing the rehabilitation of displaced tribals, sums up the situation as below :

> "The Working Group felt that absence of a national policy for rehabilitation of displaced tribals has been the chief reason for the present state of affairs. The Working Group felt that various guidelines have no doubt been issued from time to time regarding rehabilitation of the displaced persons including tribals, the latest by the Bureau of Public Enterprises 10 February, 1986. But these have remained only as pious declaration of intention and have remained on paper only.
>
> The Working Group felt that a comprehensive National Policy which will provide for complete socio-economic rehabilitation of displaced tribals, is very much required. The Working Group felt that the policy must aim at ensuring a better living standard to the displaced tribal families at the relocation sites and must be backed up by a Central Authority under a legislation for its enforce-ment. In the absence of a Central Authority for enforcing the policy, the Working Group felt, the policy may remain on paper like the guidelines issued by the various Departments/Ministries in the past".

That was in the year 1989. In the last Conference of Ministers and Secretaries of States and Union Territories concerned with tribal development organised by the Ministry of Welfare, Government of India, the current policy of the States for rehabilitation of displaced tribals was very much in the agenda. The Ministry stated that "formulation of a national policy for rehabilitation of project displaced persons belonging to Scheduled Tribes has become an imperative", as "the chief instrument for acquiring private land for public purposes (Land Acquisition Act 1894) does not provide for rehabilitation". The Ministry's note also included salient provisions that should be included in the national policy.

The Parliamentary Committee on the Welfare of Scheduled Castes and Scheduled Tribes, which is a Standing Committee have also decided to examine the issue—rehabilitation of tribals by major projects.

Non-government organisations have in recent years been playing a very important role in examining the extent of displacement, adequacy or otherwise of rehabilitation measures and the policies followed by the government departments, corporations, companies, etc. in different parts of the country. They have also been agitating for the rights of the oustees. The Narmada Bachao Andolan (Jain 1993; Nayar, 1993; Menon 1993; Mohan 1993) gave such agitations the spirit and shape of a strong movement, associating with it a number of PAPs, organizations, environmental protection organisations and people from the Sarvodaya movement. The National Working Group on Displacement have issued a draft national policy on developmental resettlement of project affected people (Fernandes and Thukral 1989; Cernea 1990). This draft is a comprehensive document spelling out the urgent need for a national policy, basic approach to development project displacement and resettlement, manner in which plans should be formulated for the development resettlement of all the PAPs, core provisions of development resettlement and the need for a national legislation including the ground which such a legislation should cover.

The Ministry of Rural Development have since prepared a revised Draft National Policy for Rehabilitation of Persons Displaced as a Consequence of Acquisition of Land, "which is expected to be the National Policy or an overriding document covering all forms of displacement" and it "can be said to reflect the thinking of the Government of India as a whole" (Fernandes 1997). According to Fernandes (*ibid*) this policy as well as other such policies have been drafted under pressure from the World Bank" and not "out of conviction". The Draft Policy itself admits reasons like: the PAPs are 'no more in a mood to accept sufferings'; 'protest movements marked by a growing militancy'; 'national awareness of the problem'; the constitutional right is affected; 'environmental concerns'; 'human rights conventions'; and 'the fact that financial institutions go to the extent of withholding loan'. Fernandes (1997) goes on to compare this Draft Policy with the 'Citizens Draft (1995)' and concludes that 'the solutions it presents leave much to be desired'. He argues for basic changes in the paradigm of our development and planning process itself to achieve a people oriented model of development.

10

FINDINGS AND SUGGESTIONS

The Study

THIS study was undertaken in the Sonbhadra district of Uttar Pradesh where large scale displacements occurred due to the construction of irrigation projects, power projects and industries. The area had a substantial (42.5%) population of tribals, and Scheduled Castes. The effect of the projects on the people in general and the tribals/ Scheduled Castes in particular which was by and large adverse has come to wider notice. Our objectives were to find out the extent of displacement and the economic base of the PAPs; the rehabilitation package admissible to them and the effectiveness of its delivery; determination of the reasons which impeded efficacy of rehabilitation; the present status of PAPs; and measures necessary for a satisfactory rehabilitations.

The study covered the rehabilitation colonies and villages inhabited by the PAPs in the areas of six projects. The projects included Rihand Dam (1960) onwards to the NCL coalfields where displacement was continuing till the time of the study (1992-93) and also the Kanhar irrigation project where land had been formally acquired but, in most cases, left with the would-be 'oustees' because work on the project was progressing very slowly due to paucity of funds. These projects were created by two giant PSUs of the Government of India, UPSEB—a

Government of U.P. enterprise, and the Irrigation Department of Uttar Pradesh. The approaches and policies guiding resettlement were found to be of a varied nature and uneven.

The study approached the PAPs at three levels—on the family level for which 1,038 schedules were canvassed, being about 10 per cent of the displaced families, in fifty-six villages/colonies; on the individual level, by collecting data for thirty-one case studies focusing on the problems and trauma of displacement and its impact on the life of these individuals; and ethnographic details concerning the different caste groups residing in their original villages. In both the case studies and family schedules, the details of rehabilitation package together with the manner in which it was delivered or managed by the authorities concerned were focal issues. The third level was the caste/tribe, for which the ethnographic accounts of the tribal and Schedule Caste groups reflected in the sample were updated in a diachronic sequence from the first decade of this century to the present time. Besides, the data available from some secondary sources were also used. These included the census data and the 'Socio-Economic Section' of the report of the Environmental Impact Assessment Study undertaken by M/s EDF International, France, on behalf of the NTPC. Prembhai of the Banwasi Sewa Ashram, Govindpur and Avadhesh of the Srajan Lokhit Samiti, Vindhyanagar (M.P.) also provided some valuable published and unpublished material. The EDF study undertaken during 1988-90 was, however, 'restricted to an area roughly surrounding the Rihand lake the totality of the small plain of Baidan (Madhya Pradesh included in it and some desert places north of Renukoot (near the Dam in Uttar Pradesh) having been excluded" (Heuze-Brigant 1991). Even though this study contains some important findings and it was initiated due to the pressure of the World Bank the NTPC have not made it public. The data thus collected brought out the present conditions among the PAPs in a comprehensive perspective.

Project's Approach to Rehabilitation

The approach of the Rihand project authorities stands out in a totally different light when compared to the later displacements. Rihand resettlement took into consideration the position that the cash compensation payable to the land-holders would be very small. Therefore, the policy of land for land and land for landless agricultural labourers as well was followed. The efforts of the oustees themselves and some help from the government succeeded in getting the PAPs integrated into the host villages around which forest/revenue land was given to them. The compensations were as low as Rs. 25-30 for a house and about Rs. 100 per *bigha* for even good-quality land. It is difficult to determine the exact number of oustees and those who got land. PAPs, obviously, could never reach the economic levels they were deprived of because the Singrauli basin area they had left was fertile while the land they got was mostly hilly and rocky and reclamation was difficult. In this connection the difficulties faced by the people on ouster, forced on them through the release of water in the reservoir during the rainy season of 1960, stands out as an act of callousness. Subsequently, many families encountered great hardships, spending more than a year in the open. Later, the government provided some facilities in the villages where they had settled on their own or were provided land. Since people were allowed to choose the area for resettlement, they moved in homogeneous groups or small communities and could thereby continue their network of intercaste relations, family ties, customary festivals and rituals alongwith their economic base of agriculture. The economic base, however, shrunk due to the absence or poor quality of forests around the new settlements and some changes in the *pati* or *jajmani* relations and reduced demands for traditionally produced items like handloom cloth and iron artifacts.

Certain assurances were given to the oustees, the foremost came from no less a person than the Late Prime Minister Nehru. He had in his speech described Rihand as 'one of the temples of modern India' and assured the people that they would be the first to get electricity which was going to be generated, and irrigation for their lands. An old person among our informants frankly said that they had then moved out of their ancestral homes without much rancour and had dreamt of better days and then bitterly complained that they had been treated in a very shabby manner and found that not even a simple assurance like supply of electricity was fulfilled. The effectiveness of the delivery of this land for land scheme of rehabilitation was, however, flawed on two counts, viz., the PAPs were in most cases, not granted a legal title or *patta* for the lands allotted to them, and there was no effort to monitor the extent of actual levels of rehabilitation. The first lacuna caused a chain of problems for the Rihand PAPs in getting compensation when they were displaced for the second and the third time and in getting loans for developing their land, while the second lacuna has been responsible for a complete absence of data relating to the quantity and quality of rehabilitation achieved, as compared to the vast number of persons displaced. In retrospect, it has also to be considered whether a dam to produce 500 MW of electricity but little irrigation facilities was worth the social cost of submerging 162 villages dotting a fertile basin and affecting a population estimated at about two lacs (EDF 1990) and 1.06 lac acres of land.

The subsequent projects started coming up after a lapse of about fifteen years. The rehabilitation approach of all these projects has the following aspects in common :

(i) There was no land for land dispensation which has meant a transformation in the economic base of the oustees.

(*ii*) Compensation was entirely in cash strictly within the framework of two laws, viz. LAA 1894 and CBAA 1957. This meant that no benefits of any kind were available to any person having no title or a weak title to the land he was cultivating or to persons who were a part of the agricultural work force through being agricultural labourers, crop-sharers, *pati*, etc.

(*iii*) While the PSUs of the Government of India gave assurances, formally or informally, in the light of guidelines of the Bureau of Public Enterprises about giving one job to each oustee family the fulfilment of the assurances was a different matter. The UPSEB controlling Anpara project also extended job assurances in the light of the fact that the Government of U.P. and its enterprises then had a policy directives to this effect. They hardly followed this up as the policy was later changed. The Irrigation Department gave no promises for jobs even though there were clear orders to that effect at that time from the Government of U.P.

(*iv*) In respect of the PAPs getting benefit of other employment or vocational opportunities through the intervention or initiative of the project authorities, again, certain assurances were given by the PSUs of the Government of India. Generally the PAPs, were at the time of take over of their lands made to believe that opportunities for a change in and a widening of their economic base would be ample once the work on the project started. The fulfilment of these assurances varied from situation to situation and at different times in the progress of the same project. In the early stages people got labour work which went on decreasing with the completion of project constructions and the tightening stranglehold of the contractors who were outsiders and their migrant labour force.

(v) A policy of providing developed plots for housing—size 60′ x 40′ or 50′ x 30′—was followed in all cases except Kanhar. The delivery of this part of the rehabilitation package was also far from satisfactory. PAPs started getting plots several years after they had physically shifted or been forced to shift from their houses and a sizeable percentage have not got plots till now.

(vi) Full development of plots and all the basic amenities in the rehabilitation colonies were unequivocally promised by all the project authorities. Here, again, the delivery of the amenities and development of colonies has been extremely tardy, the conditions varying from one colony to another—"characterized by a lack of technical know-how and inadequate resources, insufficient even for the modest objectives which had been set. The promises about schools, roads and dispensaries have rarely been kept" (EDF 1990). "The majority of these colonies are situated in locations best suited for garbage disposal rather than for accommodating human beings" (Heuze-Brigant 1991). Even an approach road with a safe railway-line crossing has been denied to Chilkadand, one of the largest rehabilitation colony, for all these fifteen years. "Families (between 4 and 25 pepole) have been allotted plots of 50′ □ 30′ and encouraged to build their houses on land which is liable to flooding (by running water, lake or ash-dumps) and/or is damp, exposed to the mosquito menace, is far

away from the city, job sites and markets, under high tension lines or located on hilly and rocky grounds in the vicinity of blasting zones" (Heuze-Brigant 1991).

(vii) The attitude of callousness and an almost inhuman approach in dealing with the PAPs was first noticed in case of Rihand itself (Commissioner 1991). Subsequently, the other project managements too have handled matters in still worse ways. Anpara oustees reported many bulldozings of their houses and ouster in the rainy season. The NTPC Bijpur, also acted similarly while the NCL emerged as topping them all. Bulldozing was noticed in several locations in January and June 1992, and some oustees employed on muster roll by the NCL were pressurised by their officers that their services would be terminated if they did not induce the people in their villages to shift. Further, the use of dynamite in close proximity of some of the rehabilitation areas or still existing parts of old villages is endangering the lives of the people and their cattle and damaging their houses. Besides what we saw, a recent report of Katiyar (1993) was equally damning.

(viii) The economic base of the PAPs has undergone a total change. Generally speaking, the extent of landlessness has become near-universal—in Singrauli area 77.4 per cent having land before displacement were reduced to 14.6 per cent, in Anpara 88 per cent land-holders were reduced to 20 per cent—and other assets like milch cattle, bullocks, fruit and timber trees, etc. have also been reduced to almost the same extent. An overwhelming majority (89.6%) of these people have no regular employment and depend only on casual wage-labour work.

Even this is not available for all the days in a month and the wages being paid by the employers like labour contractors, etc. are much below the fixed minimum wage. Impoverishment is to be seen everywhere and the people variously expressed it in words like "we have been ruined" or "we have become beggars" or "nobody is prepared to listen" to us. There is an overwhelming psychological feeling of marginalisation among the people who widely expressed their 'help-lessness' through comments like 'no one cares for us' or 'listens to us'. Their attachment with land is so overwhelming that some still go on to describe themselves as "agriculturists", though they might have lost their entire land holdings.

(ix) Large joint families which were found to be the rule in rural areas occupied by the Rihand oustees have started disintegrating into nuclear families mainly due to change in economic base. This trend has been further encouraged by the rehabilitation policy of providing small plots which are strictly of urban standards. A plot of the size of 50′ x 30′ or even 60′ x 40′ does not take care of any milch cattle, goats, etc. which these people still continue to rear. As Heuze-Brigant tersely describes, "The families are split but this is not always considered a negative event. Families are not easy to destroy. The village or the *basti* is the main casuality. Usually the villages have been relocated together in rehabilitation colonies. The problem is that a village population relocated in the rows of a rehabilitation settlement with inhospitable roads and a disgusting environment, becomes inopera-tive as a community" (1991 : 318). Our data, *inter*

alia, delineated relevant aspects of tribe-caste relations in the area and, the structure of the village communities with particular reference to the role of these relations in evolving some pattern of leadership. Analysing different aspects of the tribe-caste relationships, their levels of integration and their ability to emerge as a cohesive village community with effective leadership and potential to organise any concerted action to face desplacement and its consequences, it was observed that leadership in the villages was diffused and segmented into caste and tribal groups with no 'dominant caste' exercising its role in the village communities. This vaccum in leadership, lack of cohesion and absence of any education rendered these communities incapable of initiating any 'constitutional' or 'direct collective action' to counter or reduce the reign of terror and injustice foisted upon them, for decades. Only in the eighties when two NGOs, headed by outsiders connected with Sarvodaya, Bhoodan, etc., took up their cause a better deal for the oustees of Bijapur NTPC project was wrested.

The Present Policy

The absence of a national policy supported by a suitable legislation in our country where the displacements are enormous, has been emphasised without any exception by all those who have dealt with the subject. For want of a national policy which would naturally be treated as a normative and compulsive frame for all rehabilitation activities we had to fall back on an examination of the guidelines, executive instructions and such other instruments and also the content of the project reports. Since the projects in Sonbhadra district are being implemented by various authorities, an examination of relevant data as made in this report brings out the following salient findings :

(a) The Bureau of Public Enterprises, Government of India, oversees the working of the central PSUs and their guidelines should apply to the NCL and the NTPC projects. These guidelines are almost without any substantive directions, *inter alia*, mentioning the need to exclude valuable agricultural land from acquisition; expeditious payment of compensation; drawing up of rehabilitation schemes relating to the tribals in consultation with the Ministry of Welfare and the Ministry of Environment and Forests; monitoring of rehabilitation work by the rehabilitation cells attached to the projects; and preparation of schemes to train and educate the PAPs in the existing institutions for equipping them to take up jobs in the project or elsewhere. The most important part of these guidelines is that the obligation if any, formal or informal, for providing jobs has been totally dropped. Both the NCL and the NTPC projects in Sonbhadra district were found to have done little in pursuance of the positive guidelines. The NTPC acquired good agricultural land and the acquisition was in excess of their requirement, since they could subsequently transfer more than a thousand acre of land to the NCL and the railways making a profit of about one crore over the prices at which they had acquired it. Tardiness in payment of compensation was widespread and nowhere did we come across any training and educational programme to upgrade the skills of the PAPs, except a brief training in carpentry conducted by the NTPC

Bijpur which proved to be a non-starter. Further, there was no evidence of any coordination with the Ministry of Welfare in planning the rehabilitation programme for tribals and Scheduled Castes who live all over the area. The Rehabilitation Cells were 'monitoring' the rehabilitation in a routine manner by indicating the number of plots allotted and oustees taken in employ-ment.

(b) The guidelines issued by the nodal ministry for the welfare of Scheduled Castes/Tribes emphasises the adoption of a liberal formula for compen-sation; providing agricultural land to some extent at least so that the tribals are not uprooted from traditional occupations; pre-paration of project reports for resettlement with the help of personnel conversant with tribal culture; rehabilitation of tribals as a community; free developed housing plots; jobs when agricultural land was not given; and training programme for creating entrepreneurial skills with subsequent provision of all facilities necessary to develop alternative occupations. These guidelines can be said to have been followed by the central PSUs in respect of providing housing plots with varying quality of basic amenities and some jobs only. No resettlement plans beyond allocation of sites were drawn for the local communities and no training programmes of the kind mentioned therein have ever been initiated by any project. The projects hnd no personnel equipped to deal with tribals and their rehabilitation needs. Resettlement package or schemes were also not found to have been made an integral part of the projects.

(c) The guidelines, by and large, take into account

only the post-project situation. Any policy or strategy to comprehensively ensure benefits of industrialisation both to the PAPs as well as the affected tribal hinterlands has not been put forward; though Sharma (1975) had spelt out such a plan in the Ministry of Home Affairs and tried to build it up into the TSP, the all inclusive paradigm for tribal development initiated in mid-seventies.

(d) The guidelines of the Ministry of Home Affairs and also the Ministry of Water Resources urge the State governments to have a law on the lines of the Maharashtra Resettlement of Displaced Persons Act 1976. No such measure has been contemplated by the Government of Uttar Pradesh so far.

(e) The orders on the subject issued by the Government of Uttar Pradesh from time to time are applicable to their Irrigation Department (Rihand and Kanhar) and also to the UPSEB (Anpara and Obra) when adopted by the Board. These orders have no provision for 'land for land' resettlement. They, *inter alia*, instruct the departments to provide built-up houses and jobs. None of the projects under the Government of Uttar Pradesh have provided any built-up houses. Only Anpara provided plots while the rest provided cash compensation only. This approach is a contrast from the generous rehabilitation package provided to the Tehri Dam oustees by the Government of U.P. As regards provision of jobs, all the project authorities stated clearly that they did not follow any such policy.

The World bank have adopted a set of guidelines and operational instructions to be followed in so far as the

World Bank aided projects are concerned. These are supplemented by a special frame for introducing a tribal component in the rehabilitation policies of the projects which have tribal PAPs. In this study, the two NTPC projects were the only recipients of World Bank finance. Therefore, it was expected that these projects would include rehabilitation component based on the World Bank policy and operational frame. The Singrauli project was started in 1977 and the World Bank had not till then adopted a clear cut policy. However, the Bijpur project came up in 1982 and by that time the World Bank had formulated their policy and operational guidelines.

EDF Survey (1990) remarks that, 'NTPC rehabilitation has been realised to be poor. But now at Rihand (Bijpur) where displacement still continues competent officials seem to have decided to change the policy. They talk of a model city, bringing rehabilitation colonies into a category of official cities. Setting up of vocational training linked with the rehabilitation is also planned." However, several years after this optimistic evaluation, we found little positive evidence of the changed rehabilitation policy on the ground. There was no vocational training programme except in one instance which led to no results as no stipend or any other incentive was provided for the ten or so trainees in carpentry. The bias of the project managers came out in a brief discussion with the Deputy General Manager who thought that the people around were "not civilised", and yet, "NTPC had given so much to them".

Attitudes like this bring to fore another important issue. The World Bank operational guidelines justifiably attach importance to the planning and implementation and also evaluation of the rehabilitation package being guided by "professional sociological advice, specially when dealing with isolated or culturally non-homogeneous populations or with particulaly vulnerable groups" (Cernea 1988a). In the course of this study efforts were made to find out the organisational set up and the training/back-ground of the personnel involved in what was called 'R&R' in the projects. Nowhere it was found that any social scientist had been recruited to handle rehabilitation and resettlement. The NTPC corporate office and the Bijpur plant did not think it proper to provide any information, one wonders why? NTPC Singrauli was however, more helpful. The portfolio was in all cases with engineers at middle to top levels somewhere, for example in the NCL and the NTPC Bijpur. Some personnel management/labour welfare people were also found involved in it, but at lower levels. The NPTC corporate office at New Delhi had also treated R&R in a similar fashion. One of their Consultants was for environment but none for social planning. By and large, the personnel not only suffered from a complete ignorance of the social environment surrounding them but they also suffered from an 'engineering bias' (Cernea 1993; 1991; EDF 1990).

Furthermore, the concerned personnel were found to have become inaccessible to the common PAPs and were functioning in a kind of isolation. They functioned generally through a selected handful of 'leaders', mostly migrants to the area. The security system of high walls, well-guarded gates with issuance of passes only to those who could satisfy all queries and link their purpose to some clearly identified officer to be met, which the common PAP can never do, were the factors which prevented any interaction, understanding or rapport with the people. The EDF study, describing the township of the projects points out how these are 'cut-off' from the environment, 'occupy a considerable amount of space' which "tends to become increasingly enclosed". "The townships do not have the object of becoming incorporated with local economic life and they are almost wholly cut off from society . . . Anything which allows peasants and casual workers to survive—pasture, trading or housing—is prohibited. Further, the senior managers of the NTPC and the mines do not know the region adequately". The training of the public and private sector managers is 'almost nil regarding social issues' and 'Public sector officials do not like organised set ups (a community or village). They only want to deal with assisted individuals, especially among the oustees" (Heuze-Brigant 1991). In general, local demands are regarded as being counter-productive and tiresome. "The quasi-colonial aspect of the township is certainly exacerabated at Singrauli, because of the weakness (low level of education, poverty and lack of connections) of the people in the area". In the course of our own study we did not come across any forum which could contribute to bridging this gap and allowing any participation by the PAPs in the managements' rehabilitation effort. On the other hand the formal committees with some representation from the oustees seldom met and efforts were made to scuttle oustee participation and decisions.

The Resultant Situation

The policy frame and operational guidelines of the World Bank discussed earlier flow out of their analysis of a vast and extensive evidence coming from numerous displacements and resettlements processes. Cernea (1990a, 1990b, and 1991) presents this analysis as a 'model of impoverishment risks' or 'a taxonomy of adverse consequences'. The pattern of recurrent characteristics reveals seven dimensions of this impoverishment risk model :

Landlessness

Compensation in cash does not ensure the replacement of the lost land and the oustees remain landless for ever. Landlessness is higher for families who have only customary rights rather than formal titles for example tribal groups in India. Loss of land is the single most important cause of impoverishment. The high incidence of landlessness created by all the displacements in Sonbhadra, after Rihand Dam, has been documented by us.

Joblessness
Risk of the oustees becoming permanently jobless sometimes after displacement or after construction works drop are high. In Sonbhadra since the oustees were all agriculturists there was no question of losing any formal job. However, with the loss of land the share-croppers, agricultural labourers and the beneficiaries of the *pati* or *jajmani* all lost their 'jobs' in one go.

Homelessness
The loss of shelter through displacement is temporary for most of those displaced. But for some families it remains a permanent condition, since compensation for acquired dwellings was paid at the assessed rather than their replacement value. To quote an example from our experience—the compensation paid for a dwelling by the NCL was Rs. 147. Can the oustee now have any kind of a dwelling for his family for this amount?

Marginalization
Project affected families cannot fully restore their prior economic strength. It seems that the projects assume as a matter of course that those displaced cannot be guaranteed re-establishment at their prior standard of living. It implies that a majority of resettlers who were in the poverty group, or just above it, would face further en-masse marginalisation and impoverishment.

Morbidity
The adverse health effects of forced displacement are commonly seen. There is a higher degree of exposure to illness and to comparatively more severe and new diseases. These may be caused by poor hygienic

conditions, pollution, inadequate supply of potable water, etc. in resettlement colonies. Most of our informants emphasised that they and their families had become prone to many diseases like asthama and tuberculosis due to pollution (thermal power projects), coal dust (open pit coal mining), poor supply of potable water and similar factors. Even Rihand reservoir is now polluted with ash-dykes of the NTPC. A senior engineer of the UPSEB told us that the NTPC had fenced ash-dyke areas when the reservoir was at a low level during summer, thereby enclosing much of the land that would have been filled up with water during monsoon. Thus ash was getting washed into the reservoir. Disintegration of the traditional system of medicine due to the non-availability of competent Baigas and their herbal pharmacopoeia and absence of facilities for modern medicine in the rehabilitation areas/colonies are adding to the morbidity levels. Lokayan Evam Lokhit Samiti, M.P. has called attention to pollution of Rihand water by Hindalco, lack of potable water for casual labour in the NCL and the diseases caused by increasing flesh-trade (Setu 1985).

Food Insecurity

Uprooting increases the risk that larger number of people will fall into the strata affected by chronic food insecurity, defined as calorie-protein intake levels, due to discontinuation of food production by themselves, decrease in purchasing power and non-availability of food stuffs at reasonable price. Our informants universally complained of their inability to get adequate food due to their poor incomes and high prices, absence of fairprice shops under public distribution system in rehabilitation colonies and the gradual disappearance of forests and restrictions on their access to the forests from where they were obtaining several items of nutritious diet and herbal medicines.

Social Disarticulation

This aspect of impoverishment is not so patent and yet it commands a great disturbing force. It may include distur-bance or disintegration of kinship and social networks, breakup of authority systems, loss of leadership and mutual help, etc. These had provided the oustees in the past with production-oriented organisations, stable marriage and ritual arrangements and other kinds of support and guidance. Our study brought forth many dimensions of this loss of network and other impondera-biliaty—unpouderabilia of culture with serious consequences for the oustees. Further, the feeling of powerlessness, alienation and even disorientation was found to be overwhelming among the oustees at all the three levels—individual, family and community (tribe/caste).

Concluding Discussion

We cannot but agree with Cernea (1990) that "impoverishment is not inevitable" . . . and the "theoretical possibility to take policy and programme actions that could counter the risks" is very much there. "But failure to recognise the risks *inherent* along these lines will allow such risks to unfold unimpeded, causing pervasive im-poverishment" and this is exactly what is happening in Sonbhadra, as per our observations. "In the rehabilitation colonies, people who cooperated with one another yesterday have no reason to do so when agriculture is dead and where competition has become the slogan of the times. It is a good case for endless quarrels around the water points. . ." (Heuze-Brigant 1991). Continuing with the argument that the adverse impact of forced displace-ment can be considerably mitigated, Cernea (1990) spells out a change in the approach to the planning and execution of the programme to achieve this objective. The adoption of "four inter-related frameworks required for involuntary settlement—policy, legal, planning and organisational—can mitigate to a large extent the adverse effects.

We have already discussed the absence of a national policy on resettlement and the present policy scenario in respect of the agencies responsible for the projects studied in Sonbhadra. It has been pointed out that the NTPC have hardly followed the BPE guidelines or the World Bank's directions and operational guidelines. The NCL too have got a rather knee-jerk approach to rehabilitation and resettlement using strong-arm methods and cosmetic measures to assuage the PAPs, alternately. Then, the Irrigation Department of the Government of Uttar Pradesh has followed a discriminatory policy—compare the resettlement package for the Tehri Dam Project and for Kanhar, and UPSEB, a Government of U.P. enterprise has no rehabilitation policy worth the name.

The legal frame work was also examined and the LAA 1894 which provides for cash compensation only to those having 'interest' in the land were found to be inequitable, inadequate and archaic in its approach. In the context of Sonbhadra, these deficiencies were found to be further exacerbated because of disputed and infirm titles of the tillers to their lands and the absence of a free market selling of land in the context of its history as a Partially Excluded Area. In this context the weakness of the PAPs to properly present and pursue their cause due to illiteracy, backwardness, lack of leadership and a general attitude of submissiveness to authority was also noted. The efforts of the NGOs towards fighting for equitable compensation and additional rehabilitation facilities have also been described but it must be said that both the district authorities and project managements have been successful in preventing any NGO organised by the oustees to take roots.

The third framework is of planning proper resettlement programmes. Discussing this aspect Cernea (1991) emphasizes that "Even in countries where policy framework exists, national agencies only rarely possess the skilled staff needed for resettlement. Social planning skills must be brought into the early preparation of resettlement projects. Anthropological and sociological resettlement expertise is necessary to design resettlement operations so that they are compatible with the resettlers' and hosts' socio-cultural institutions". The five main components in the planning framework for displacement and resettlement spelt out by Cernea (1991)—(i) development 'packages' and alternative options; (ii) compensation; (iii) new habitat; (iv) the social organisation of resettlers; and (v) the host population and the environmental protection of the relocation area—were all conspicuous by their absence in Sonbhadra. Cernea (1990) specificially mentions India as one of the countries where, "lessons derived from dam-related dislocations show that it is necessary to examine the situation of each socio-economic category of the displaced population whether land holders or landless employees or artisans, to ensure that options are available to them in a comprehensive programme of resettlement". The 'development packages' must offer sufficient opportunities and resources for their economic and social re-establishment as self sustaining producers or wage-earners.

Similar instructions are contained in the guidelines issued for Scheduled Caste/Tribe PAPs both by the BPE and the nodal Ministry. While India has no dearh of the kind of skilled persons needed for resettlement work it was found that there were hardly any such persons in the set-up looking after R&R in the projects and, further, no advance or even contemporary exercise in this direction had been undertaken. The projects had no baseline data like socio-economic profile of the PAPs, their cultural institutions, inter and intra-caste/tribe network and other institutions. Whatever was offered, for instance housing plots in rehabilitation colonies, was found to be incompatible with the PAPs pattern of life and its delivery was tardy and without the much needed human touch. The owners of houses bull-dozed by the NCL were assured a payment of Rs. 10,000 each which had still not come and the affected persons were living under the trees. Other agencies like the district administration, involved in rehabilitation, also suffered from the same deficiencies. Participation of the PAPs in the planning process was nearly absent. They were usually not taken into confidence and when their representatives were associated, some assurances—like providing one job to each family and economic opportunities through other channels—were voiced before them which warped the judgements of such representatives. For instance, it was claimed that an offer was made to the NTPC/NCL oustees around Chilkadand to settle down on land in Ghorawal block. The PAPs, however, refused going to such a far off place. We were informed that these people were kept under the impression that there would be jobs, one for each family (an assurance which the BPE policy ruled out) and therefore they did not agree to move. But was this offer a full 'package' at all?

The case of Narmada Dam Projects which have displaced and continue to displace tribal communities in very large numbers has now become quite well known. What has been concluded about the resettlement plans for the affected area by Morse (1992 : 349-52) further confirms our observations. In the context of Narmada Project in Gujarat, Joshi (1987) has classified the impact which the displacements would make into three geographical zones, depending on the level of acculturation of the tribal communities and their socio-economic interests. It is likely that such differentiations into geographical zones can be seen in the areas to be affected by the Narmada Project which are vast, but we have to take into account the fact that in the Narmada project affected areas preparation and planning for displacement have been going on for decades and this has contributed to the preparedness of the oustees and also the preparation of systematic relo-cation and resettlement plans as documented by Verma (1985). Yet, it made Morse to observe that the record of resettlement and rehabilitation in India, "has been unsatis-factory in virtually every project, with a large resettlement component . . ." (1992 : 351). In contrast, the Sonbhadra oustees were destined to face sudden jolts of displacements, more than one in the case of a substantial population, without any advance planning for their economic and social rehabilitation or even a sound policy in that direction. Here, nearly "all the communities, tribal or non-tribal endure almost the same process of alienation and dispossession" (Heuze-Brigant 1989), as the villages in the area were characterised by a lack of sharp differences in the economic strata of the people and the absence of any assertive leadership which might have helped in getting a better deal and enabled them to create organisations to pursue their aims, unlike the Narmada Project and Tehri Dam PAPs. This is well explained through the characteristics of 'fringe villages' by Majumdar (1960). The homogeneity and egalitarian outlook of the people, with little feudalistic shades, can prove helpful in forging a unity of response from them to any alternative plan for their rehabilitation and resettlement which is being suggested here.

Joshi (1987) found that in the tribal villages of Gujarat, studied by him, the differential attitudes towards the issue of rehabilitation among the interest groups in the villages were marked and the would-be oustees were found to be divided on the lines of educated large land-holders and comparatively small farmers belonging to different sections of the Tadavi tribe. He, therefore, cautions against rehabilitation policy and programme "based on the narrow concept of shifting the households from one locality to other", and rightly points out that "rehabilitation should be redefined as grafting a community at a new place and nurturing it to ensure its steady and balanced growth". A self-standing programme of shifting should be of such a nature and the sociological characteristics of the Sonbhadra PAPs seem to be such that this strategy is likely to yield encouraging results, once the people are disabused of the notion that projects could employ all the young men and then revive their shaken faith in the administration and project managements. Of course the families who have either obtained regular jobs or settled themselves by making judicious investment of the compensation would not be enthusiastic about shifting to agriculture base in some other areas.

Suggestions

The most important objective of this study was to suggest measures that need to be taken in order to make rehabilitation successful and more effective in Sonbhadra. Our empirical data and review and analysis of secondary data has thrown a good deal of light on the prevailing scenario and the kind of difficulties the PAPs are facing. But practical corrective measures in order to achieve durable rehabilitation can be thought of in a long term perspective only while some relief and succour can be provided in the colonies straightaway.

Preparing the Data Base

The most essential aspect that has to be tackled is the creation of a well coordinated set up to make a comprehensive study of the present needs of the oustees and a data base to plan alternative strategies for rehabilitation. This has to be done by appropriate personnel having a knowledge of the cultural configurations and potentialities of the people and the area. Actual participation of the representatives of the oustees from rehabilitation areas and the NGOs who have the necessary experience has to be ensured in the work. With this data base, rehabilitation plans have to be prepared for the different groups namely persons having skills in agricultural work, forest work, cattle keeping, pisci-culture, technical (artisans) and those engaged in such other work. This plan can be subsumed under two strategies—land based strategies and non-land based strategies.

Relocation in Agriculature

A majority of the PAPs were still oriented to homogeneous community living with moorings in their old villages. Therefore, they can move in such groups to areas where land can be found for them to restart agricultural operations. Some areas in the district, such as the stretch north-west of Bijpur upto the Kanhar command area in Dudhi, can be available for creating resettlement villages as full, free-standing projects on their own. The district still has a low population density and natural resource bases for agriculture abound as pointed out earlier in this report. Cernea (1990) mentions the success of such projects in Mexico and, nearer home, resettlement on this pattern has been taken up for Narmada project oustees. The amendments to LAA 1894 made by Uttar Pradesh include a provision for acquiring land for allocation to landless persons and the comprehensive Maharashtra law is already there as a model. Such projects would accommodate substantial numbers of oustees who had an agricultural-based economy and still prefer it. The projects will have to include a complete package: land, its reclaimation, development and other investments as well as sustenance amounts to the settlers' families. If the Government of U.P. could do it for the Tehri oustees and for Sikh settlers and agriculture graduates in the Tarai area the Sonbhadra PAPs deserve it the most, by way of an act of restoring their human and constitutional rights and dignity. The World Bank also extends assistance for such projects.

Non-agricultural Pursuits

Alternatively, for a family or group of families of oustees who can take up dairying on a viable basis the best location would be around the project colonies and other semi-urban conglomerations where the demand for dairy products is good and fast going up. Our data disclosed that under the Integrated Rural Development Programme and/or Special Component Plan for Scheduled Castes a very small number of our respondents had taken benefit of loans for milch cattle. Most of those who had taken up such a scheme reported death of buffaloes/cows they had purchased. The experience from the IRDP scheme has been that the funding for milch cattle was inadequate and even the amount sanctioned for purchasing cows/ buffaloes was partly absorbed by a whole chain of corrupt functionaries in the banks and the blocks. Therefore, the dairy projects for PAPs will need a different set of norms and adequate funding through cooperatives or NGOs together with allotment of suitable areas for stall-feeding and cattle movement so that the projects can be viable.

Another land-based activity which can rehabilitate PAPs is pisciculture. It is an irony that the people who lost their villages in Rihand reservoir are not entitled to fishing in this reservoir, contracts for which are given to outsiders. This approach has to be modified and tribals and other caste groups like Kewat and Kahar, who were earlier engaged in fishing as a subsidiary part of their economic base will have to be organised into cooperatives or goups to take to pisciculture as a vocation. Verma (1985) has included comprehensive scheme models for several land-based activities and also other alternative vocations.

Labour Contracts

Our data profusely documents the oustees' complaints

about the projects' labour work being contracted to outsiders who bring in migrant labour, often tribals from other states, who are treated more or less as captive labour and paid wages much lower than the prescribed minimum wage. This policy has got to be modified and adequate numbers of oustees have to be identified and organised into labour cooperative societies who should be assigned the contracts, instead of labour contractors from outside.

Business

Similarly, there is the question of providing shops, kiosks and hawking permission to cater to the needs of project areas. The guidelines of the Bureau of Public Enterprises and Ministry of Home Affairs are quite clear. The projects will have to shoulder the responsibility of making such opportunities available only to the PAPs.

Habitations

Simultaneously with the exercise of identifying PAPs needs and relating their communities/groups to different strategy alternatives the replanning or rehabilitation colonies and upgrading of the basic facilities therein has also to be given full attention. It is clear that the projects have totally failed to meet even this minimum commitment of theirs and hence they must be made responsible for remedying it.

Managing the Rehabilitation

The dimensions of the problem in Sonbhadra deserve that an authority with the necessary powers and budgetary provisions should be set up for rehabilitation and resettle-ment work. This authority can either be a part of the state directorate of rehabilitation and resettlement (Maharashtra pattern) if the U.P. government plans such a state-level body or it can be created solely for Sonbhadra through suitable legislative and executive action. In fact the latter course is more likely to yield results. This authority can be called the Authority for Sonbhadra Rehabilitation Areas (ASRA). This set-up will have to recruit personnel with the necessary skills to make the rehabilitation and resettlement package a success. The Central Government and the Government of Uttar Pradesh both have to apply themselves seriously and with a political and bureaucratic will to modify the policy frame for rehabilitation. The policy frame should not allow inequitable and differential treatment of the oustees by different projects at different places. An adequate administrative machinery and supportive laws are necessary for implementing this frame. ASRA should also have a legal aid wing to help the PAPs in settling their oustanding matters relating to compensation, further acquisitions if any, and related legal matters.

Cernea (1990, 1993) cautions about population relocation turning into implementation disasters due to the absence of distinct organisational framework for the purpose, competent staffing and commensurate resources. The organisational framework should also provide institutional arrangements for monitoring and ongoing evaluation of the dislocation and resettlement process. But this work should not be put under the direct authority of those responsible for resettlement operations. In recent years social scientists have built up a whole range of methodology and research tools for monitoring and quick evaluations (Cochrane 1979) and the ASRA will have to incorporate concurrent evaluation and monitoring through social scientists under the auspices of NGOs as a standing wing to its activities.

Policy & Legal Provisions

The application of LAA 1894 to all kinds of acquisition should be circumscribed and a rational way to amend the compensation law so as to apply it differentially—taking into account the economically stratified oustees of ours (Singh 1989). Statutory provisions would also be needed to cut down the time taken in the disposal of claims and payments of compensation and putting restraints on the government or project authorities creating all kinds of technicalities which encourage litigation and cause harassment to the poor people. The National Human Rights Commission, taking note of this area, can push through a policy and legal farme which does not overlook the individual and collective rights of the PAPs, particularly the scheduled comunities (Saksena 1995; Ali 1995). Further, in Sonbhadra the directions given by the apex court to NTPC Bijpur have created a land mark and the government and projects should, *suo motu*, initiate applying these directives to other projects, *mutatis mutandis*.

Scheduled Tribe Status

The socio-cultural status of the tribal groups is such that they deserve to be listed as Scheduled Tribes. The Government of Uttar Pradesh had recommended it long ago and have reaffirmed this stand by treating these communities as 'non-scheduled tribes' and taking up special schemes for their benefit. The Joint Committee of the Parliament headed by Chanda (Lok Sabha 1969) had also agreed to the State Government's views in so far as the tribals of Sonbhadra and the adjoining districts of the south-eastern Uttar Pradesh are concerned. Therefore, the Government of India should be responsive enough to take up without any delay the legislative move to correct the situation in Uttar Pradesh, delinking the matter from the revision of the lists of scheduled castes and scheduled tribes on a pan-Indian basis, which has remained pending due to issues not at all connected with the Uttar Pradesh proposals. Such legislative action has been taken by the Government of India recently in respect of some other States. The status of Scheduled Tribe for these people will surely provide them the benefit of a protective framework and a better and systematically planned developmental deal under the tribal sub-plan. This change would certainly help to improve and modify rehabilitation and resettlement policies and their implementation, duly supplemented by a much larger programme for the sub-plan area develop-ment and family based schemes.

The last two reports of Commissioner for Scheduled Castes and Tribes, the report of the FDF which the NTPC has held back from the public eye obviously because it is quite critical and the data put forth in our study all make it evident that the people of the area being industrialised in Sonbhadra district, including a substantial number of tribals, Scheduled Castes and weaker sections are facing acute deprivation. They have had more than their shares of grief and tears in this process of country's development. "In Singrauli progress is presently equated by the people with displacement and annihilation of local democracy" (Heuze-Brigant 1991); and the tribals, 'by nature of their physical, economic and cultural remoteness require special treatment...' (Morse 1992 : 66). A time has now come that concerted plans should be initiated for giving them a fair deal, in tune with Nehru's Tribal Panchseel (Nehru 1957).

BIBLIOGRAPHY

Adhikary, A.K. and R.K. Bhattacharya, 1982 : The Extremist Movement : An Appraisal of the Naxalite Movement with Special reference to its Repurcussions among Tribes. In K.S. Singh (ed.), *Tribal Movements in India*, Vol. 2. New Delhi: Manohar Publications.

Ali, Shaukat, 1995, *Displace Persons and Human Rights*. Paper presented at the National Seminar on Human Rights, Development and Democracy, Law School, Banaras Hindu University, March 29-31.

Baboo, Balgovind, 1993 : *Technology and Social Transformation—The Case of the Hirakud Multi-purpose Dam Project in Orissa*. Delhi: Concept Publishing Co.

B.A.J.S.S., 1951 : *Acts and Orders of the Government of India*. Delhi: Bharatiya Adimjati Sevak Sangh.

Baxi, Upendra, 1989 : Notes on Constitutional and Legal Aspects of Rehabilitation and Displacement. In Walter Fernandes and E.G. Thukral (eds.), *Development Displacement and Rehabilitation*. New Delhi: Indian Social Institute.

Bhartari, R. and A.K. Kothari, 1984 : Narmada Valley Project: Development or Destruction. *Economic and Political Weekly*, Vol. 21, No. 24.

Bebel, B.L., 1990 : *The Law Relating to Forest and Wild Life Protection* (in Hindi). Lucknow: Eastern Book Co.

Census of India, 1971 : *Series 21—Uttar Pradesh District Census Handbook—Mirzapur District Part XA—Town and Village Directory*. Lucknow: Director of Census Operations.

Census of India, 1981 : *Series—21 Part XA Town and*

Village Directory, Mirzapur District. Lucknow: Director of Census Operations.

Census of India, 1981 : *Series—22 Part XIIIB Primary Census Abstracts—District Mirzapur*. Lucknow: Director of Census Operations.

Census of India, 1981 : *Series—22 Uttar Pradesh-Paper 2 of 1982*. Lucknow: Director of Census Operations.

Cernea, Michael, M., 1988a : *Involuntary Resettlement in Development Projects: Policy Guidelines in World Bank Financed Projects*. Washington, D.C.: The World Bank.

Cernea, Michael, M., 1988b : Involuntary Resettlement and Development. *Finance and Development*, September 1988.

Cernea, Michael, M., 1990 : *Poverty Risks from Population Displacement in Water Resources Development*. Development Discussion Paper No. 355. Cambridge, Mass: Harvard University.

Cernea, Michael, M., 1991a : *Putting People First—Sociological Variables in Rural Development*. New York: Oxford University Press.

Cernea, Michael, M., 1991b : Socio-Economic and Cultural Approaches to Involuntary Population Resettlement. *Guidelines on Lake Management*. Vol. II. World Bank Reprint Series 468.

Chaudhary, S.K., 1993 : *Myopic Development and Cultural Lens : An Evaluative Study of Development Programme Among Kondhs of Orissa*. New Delhi: Inter-India Publications.

Cochrane, Glynn, 1979 : *The Cultural Appraisal of Development Projects*. New York: Praeger Publishers.

Commissioner for Scheduled Castes & Scheduled Tribes, 1988: Twentyeighth Report—1986-87. New Delhi : Manager of Publications.

Commissioner for Scheduled Castes & Scheduled Tribes, 1990: Twentyninth Report–1987-89. New Delhi: Manager of Publications.

Dhagamwar, V, 1989 : Rehabilitation Policy and

Institutional Changes Required. In Walter Fernandes and E.G. Thukral (ed.), *Development Displacement and Rehabilitation*. New Delhi: Indian Social Institute.

Drake-Brockman, D.L., 1911 : *Mirzapur. A Gazetteer*, Vol. XXVII of the District Gazetters of the United Provinces of Agra and Oudh. Allahabad: Government Press.

EDF, France, 1990 : *Report of an Environmental Impact Assessment*. New Delhi: National Thermal Power Corporation (Unpublished).

Fernandes, W. and E.G. Thukral (ed.), 1989 : *Development Displacement and Rehabilitation*. New Delhi: Indian Social Institute.

Fernandes, W., 1997: The Draft National Policy for the Rehabilitation of DPS: Is Displacement Inevitable. In W. Fernandes and V. Paranjpye (eds.) *Rehabilitation Policy and Law in India: A Right to Livelihood*. New Delhi : Indian Social Institute and ECONET.

Fernandes, W. and S. Anthony Raj, 1992 : *Development Displacement and Rehabilitation in Tribal Areas of Orissa*. New Delhi: Indian Social Institute.

Fernandes, W. (ed.), 1992 : *National Development and Tribal Deprivation*. New Delhi: Indian Social Institute.

Gupta, A., 1993 : The Other Option, *Sunday*, 15-21 August.

Hasan, Amir, 1982 : *Meet the U.P. Tribes*. Gurgaon: The Academic Press.

Hasan, Amir, 1985 : *Tribal Administration in Uttar Pradesh Since Independence*. Thesis submitted in the Department of Public Administration, Lucknow University, Lucknow.

Hasan, Amir, 1988 : *Tribal Administration in India*. Delhi: B.R. Publishing Corporation.

Heuze-Brigant, G., 1991 : Singrauli Super Thermal Project: Heavy Investment and Social Havoc, *Social Action*. 41: 3 July-September 1991.

India, Government of, 1948 : *Draft Constitution of India: Prepared by the Drafting Committee*. New Delhi:

Constituent Assembly of India.

India, Government of, 1989 : *Constitution of India*. (Seventh Edition). Lucknow: Eastern Book Co.

India, Government of, 1989 : *Report of the Working Group on Development and Welfare of Scheduled Tribes During VIII Five Year Plan*. New Delhi : Planning Commission.

India, Government of, *The Coal Bearing Areas (Acquisition and Development Act, 1957*, A.I.R. Manual, Vol. VI. Bombay: The All India Reporter Ltd.

India, Government of, 1962 : *Report of the Scheduled Area and Scheduled Tribes Commission*, Vol. I. New Delhi: Manager of Publications.

India, Government of, 1984 : *Selected Statistics on Scheduled Castes*. New Delhi: Ministry of Home Affairs.

India, Government of, 1993 : *India 1992—A Reference Annual*. New Delhi: Publications Division, India.

India, Government of, 1993 : *Land Acquisition Act, 1894*. Lucknow: Eastern Book Co.

India, Government of, 1986 : *Report of the Study Group on Land Holding Systems in Tribal Areas*. New Delhi: Planning Commission (Mimeographed).

Katiyar, Arun, 1993 : Refugees of Progress, *India Today*, September 30, 1993.

Lok Sabha, 1969 : *Report of the Joint Committee on the Scheduled Castes and Scheduled Tribes Orders (Amendment) Bill 1967*. New Delhi: Lok Sabha Secretariat.

Madge, John, 1963 : *The Tools of Social Sciences.*, London: Longmans Green and Co. Ltd.

Mahapatra, L.K., 1991 : Development for Whom? Depriving the Dispossessed Tribals, *Social Action*, 41:3.

Majumdar, D.N., 1944 : *The Fortunes of Primitive Tribes*. Lucknow: Universal Publishers, Ltd.

Majumdar, D.N., 1951 : *Races and Cultures of India*. Lucknow: Universal Publishers Ltd. (4th Revised and Enlarged Edition).

Majumdar, D.N., 1960 : *Chhor Ka Ek Gaon* (Hindi). New

Delhi : Asia Publishing House.

Mendelsohn, O. and Upendra Baxi (eds.), 1994 : *The Rights of Subordinated Peoples*. New Delhi: Oxford University Press.

Menon, M., 1993 : Dam Spells Doom for Tribals in Madhya Pradesh, *Times of India*, 6 July.

Mishra, P., 1988 : *Uttar Pradesh District Gazetteers : Mirzapur*. Lucknow: Department of District Gazetteers, U.P.

Mohan, Surendra, 1993 : Vikas Ki Disha, *Amar Ujala* (Hindi), 16 June.

Morse, B. and Berger, T., 1992 : *Sardar Sarovar : The Report of the Independent Group*. Ottawa: Resource Futures International (RFL) Inc.

Multiple Action Research Group (MARG), 1990 : *The Land Acquisition Act and You*. New Delhi.

Muthiah, S. (ed.), 1982 : *A Social and Economic Atlas of India*. Delhi: Oxford University Press.

National Institute of Rural Development, 1991 : *Rural Development Statistics—1990*. Hyderabad: NIRD.

National Thermal Power Corporation (NTPC), 1993 : *India—NTPC Rehabilitation and Resettlement Policy*, New Delhi: NTPC.

Nayar, R., 1993 : Date-line Manibeli, *Sunday*, 15-21 August.

Nehru, J., 1959 : Foreword to the Second Edition of V. Elwin's *A Philosophy for NEFA*. Shillong: North East Frontier Agency.

Patnaik, S.M., 1989 : Development and Displacement: An Analysis of Rehabilitation Policies and Programmes of Upper Kolab River Project, Orissa: *Indian Anthropologist*, Vol. 19, No. 1 & 2.

Patnaik, S.M., 1990 : Relevance of Case Study Method in Anthropology of Development, *Indian Anthropologist*, Vol. 20, No. 1 & 2.

Prembhai, Multiple Displacement and Problems of Rehabilitation in Mirzapur Tribal Area (Published

Paper).

Rao, B. Shiva (ed.), 1968 : *The Framing of India's Constitution—A Study*. New Delhi: The Indian Institute of Public Administration.

Roy Burman, B.K., 1992 : Historical Process in Respect of Communal Land System and Poverty Alleviation Among Tribes. In Walter Fernandes (ed.) *National Development and Tribal Development*. New Delhi: Indian Social Institute.

Roy B.K. and R.K. Srivastava, 1986 : *Dialogues on Development: The Individual Society and Political Order*. New Delhi.

Saksena, H.S., 1981 : *Safeguards for Scheduled Castes and Tribes—Founding Fathers, View*. New Delhi: Uppal Publishing House.

Saksena, H.S., 1995: *Human Rights and Development Caused Displacements*. Paper presented at the National Seminar on Human Rights, Development and Democracy, Law School, Banaras Hindu University, March 29-31.

SETU, 1985 : *Vikas Ki Keemat—Singrauli Mein Visthapan Ki Samasya* (Hindi). Ahmedabad: Centre for Social Knowledge and Action (SETU).

Sharma, B.D., 1975 : *Planning for Industrial Development of the Tribal Areas:* New Delhi: Government of India, Ministry of Home Affairs.

Singh, Chhatrapati, 1989 : Rehabilitation and the Right to Property. In Walter Fernandes and E.G. Thukral (eds.), *Development Displacement and Rehabilitation*. New Delhi: Indian Social Institute.

Singh, K.S., 1982 : *Tribal Movements in India,* Vol. 2. New Delhi: Manohar Publications.

Sorabjee, S., 1995: Right to Shelter is a Basic Right *The Pioneer* (Lucknow), March 21.

Tiwari, S.K., 1984 : *Madhya Pradesh Ke Adivasi* (Hindi). Bhopal: Madhya Pradesh Hindi Granth Akadmi.

U.P. Government, 1983 : *Report of the High Level Committee on the Status of Land Records and Entries Under Varg-4 in the Area South of Kaimur*. Lucknow: Department of Revenue.

U.P. Government, 1986 : *Agricultural Census in Uttar Pradesh, 1980-81*. Lucknow: Board of Revenue.

U.P. Government, 1987 : *A Hand Book of U.P. State Enterprises*. Lucknow: Sarvajanik Udyam Bureau, U.P.

U.P. Government, 1988 : *Sankhyakiya Patrika—Janpad Mirzapur* (Hindi). Lucknow: Planning Institute, U.P.

U.P. Government, 1989 : *Special Component Plan Ke Twarit evam Labhkari Karyanavan Hetu U.P. Shashan Dwara Jari Adeshon Ka Sankalan* (Hindi). Lucknow: U.P. Anusuchit Jati Vitta Evam Vikas Nigam Ltd.

U.P. Government, 1991 : *Aaudyogik Nirdeshika* (Hindi). Robertsganj: Sonbhadra District Industries Centre.

U.P. Government, 1991 : *Rajaswa Vibhag Ke Pramukh Shasanadeshon Ka Samkalan* (Hindi), (Chaturtha Khand). Lucknow: Rajaswa Vibhag.

U.P. Government of, 1992a : *Sankhyikia Patrika—Janpad Sonbhadra* (Hindi). Lucknow: State Planning Institute, U.P.

U.P. Government of, 1992b : *Sankhyikia Diary—Uttar Pradesh* (Hindi). Lucknow: State Planning Institute, U.P.

U.P. Government of, 1992c : *Uttar Pradesh Mein Samaj Kalyan Pragati Pustika—1991-2* (Hindi). Lucknow: Directorate of Social Welfare, U.P.

Verma, S.C., 1985 : *Human Settlement in Lower Narmada Basin*. Bhopal: Narmada Valley Project Authority, M.P.

Verma, Ravindra and Prembhai, 1987 : *Land Problems and the Tribal Unrest in South Mirzapur (U.P.)* (Memeographed).

INDEX